Progress in Endocrine Research and Therapy
Volume 4

INSULIN ACTION AND DIABETES

Contributors to the International Conference on Insulin Action and Diabetes

March 26–27, 1987

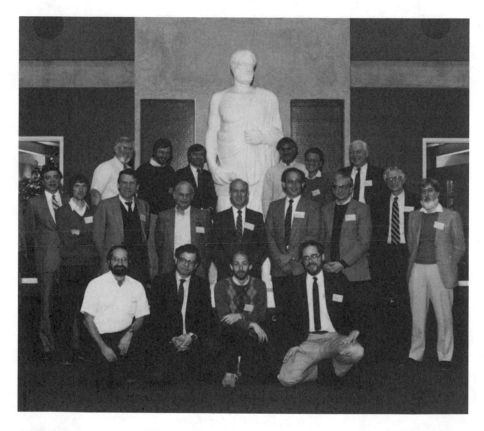

Left to right: *Back row:* Sam Cushman, Paul Pilch, Mike Czech, Ron Kahn, Cecil Yip, Charles Hollenberg. *Middle row:* Dan Roncari, Roger Brownsey, Dietrich Brandenburg, Ken Zierler, Joe Goren, Gary Friedenberg, Joe Avruch, Phil Gorden, Morley Hollenberg. *Front row:* Richard Roth, Barry Posner, Jeff Pessin, Howard Haspel.

Missing: Bill Rutter, Victoria Knutson, Hans Tornqvist, Chuck Burrant, Len Jarett, Jose Goldman, Theresa Walker, Hans Joost, Dan Lane, Ruthann Masaracchia, Ed Ryan, Gerald van de Werve, George Fantus, Richard Bergman, David Lau, Dinkar Sahal, Yan Kwok, Richard Whitesell, Amira Klip, Fred Kiechle, Elwood Walls, Yoram Shechter, Victor Garcia, Victor Lavis, Ivan Bihler, Diane Finegood, Henry Koopmans.

Progress in Endocrine Research and Therapy
Volume 4

Insulin Action and Diabetes

Editors

H. Joseph Goren, Ph.D.
*Professor, Department of
Medical Biochemistry, and
The Julia McFarlane Diabetes
Reseach Unit
Faculty of Medicine
University of Calgary
Calgary, Alberta, Canada*

Morley D. Hollenberg, D.Phil., M.D.
*Professor and Head, Department of
Pharmacology and Therapeutics, and
The Julia McFarlane Diabetes
Research Unit
Faculty of Medicine
University of Calgary
Calgary, Alberta, Canada*

Daniel A. K. Roncari, M.D., Ph.D.
*Julia McFarlane Professor of Diabetes Research,
Departments of Medicine and Medical Biochemistry
Faculty of Medicine
University of Calgary
Calgary, Alberta, Canada*

Raven Press ☙ New York

Raven Press, 1185 Avenue of the Americas, New York, New York 10036

Made in the United States of America

Library of Congress Cataloging-in-Publication Data

International Conference on Insulin Action and
    Diabetes (1987 : Calgary, Alta.)
    Insulin action and diabetes.

    (Progress in endocrine research and therapy; v. 4)
    "International Conference on Insulin Action and
Diabetes, March 26–27, 1987"—P. facing t.p.
    Includes bibliographies and index.
    1. Insulin—Physiological effect—Congresses.
2. Insulin—Receptors—Congresses. 3. Diabetes—
Pathophysiology—Congresses. I. Goren, H. Joseph.
II. Hollenberg, Morley D., 1942–   . III. Roncari,
Daniel A. K. IV. Title. V. Series. [DNLM:
1. Diabetes Mellitus—metabolism—congresses.
2. Insulin—physiology—congresses. W1 PR668QM v.4 /
WK820 I599i 1987]
RC661.I6I588   1987   616.462061   87 42837
ISBN 0-88167-448-6

The material contained in this volume was submitted as previously unpublished material, except in the instances in which credit has been given to the source from which some of the illustrative material was derived.

Great care has been taken to maintain the accuracy of the information contained in the volume. However, neither Raven Press nor the editors can be held responsible for errors or for any consequences arising from the use of the information contained herein.

9   8   7   6   5   4   3   2   1

Progress in Endocrine Research and Therapy

Preface

Probably no other hormone has received the amount of attention as has insulin. However, after some 60 years of research and four Nobel Prizes for investigations dealing with insulin, we still do not understand how insulin acts. Nonetheless, the pace of research on insulin action and diabetes has just taken a quantum jump, with the elucidation of the primary structure of the insulin receptor; questions related to the structure and function of the insulin receptor can now be addressed. Thus, in the fall of 1985, some months after the primary structure had been reported, at a meeting of the Julia McFarlane Diabetes Research Unit, it was decided to organize a Conference on Insulin Action and Diabetes in March of 1987. The main aim of the Conference was to bring together scientists with diverse interests in insulin action and diabetes, in a forum that would facilitate small group interactions that could generate new research directions.

We were delighted by the response of invited participants, and are most grateful to those who, in addition to presenting their work, provided a written account of their talks. The excitement generated by all the participants at the Conference had a positive impact on diabetes-related research in Calgary and hopefully had a similar impact on the home institutions of the participants. We hope that the publication of this Volume will help to convey the same kind of excitement to other centres of diabetes research.

This book is divided into 3 sections: Insulin Receptor, Insulin Action, and Disorders of Insulin Action. The contributions in this book illustrate the value of an integrated approach to the problem of diabetes. The breadth of the methods of investigation that were used by the contributors to this volume are most impressive and include: chemical, biochemical, molecular biological, immunological, physiological, and pharmacological. Research in 'Insulin Action and Diabetes' is ready for another quantum leap. We hope this volume may provide the necessary spring-board.

This book will be of interest to all those (clinicians, basic scientists, medical students, and graduate students) working directly in diabetes-related areas. The information will be of value to those working on mechanisms whereby a transmembrane signal is generated in response to an extracellular signal.

H. J. Goren
M. D. Hollenberg
D. A. K. Roncari

Acknowledgments

The International Conference on Insulin Action and Diabetes and the publication of this volume were sponsored in large part by the Alberta Heritage Foundation for Medical Research and The Julia McFarlane Diabetes Research Unit. Generous financial support was also provided by The American Cyanamid Corporation, Ames Limited, Ayerst Laboratories Research, Boehringer-Mannheim, Connaught-Novo Limited, Dupont Canada, The Eli Lilly Company, ICI Pharma Limited, Mandel Scientific, McNeil Pharmaceutical Company, Nordisk, and Pfizer Central Research. In addition, the Organizing Committee gratefully acknowledges the following individuals without whose efforts the Conference and the publication of its proceedings would not have occurred: Margaret-Ann Stroh of The University of Calgary Conference Office; Carol Hyman for typing the oral presentations; and Marilyn Devlin for providing excellent secretarial assistance over the past two years.

Contents

Insulin Action

Disorders of Insulin Action

Plenary Lecture

Summary

Contributors

D. Ambrosius
Deutches Wollforschungsinstitut an der
  Technischen
Hochschule Aachen
D-51 Aachen, FRG

Richard Arakaki
Diabetes Branch
National Institute of Diabetes and
  Digestive and Kidney Diseases
National Institutes of Health
Bethesda, Maryland 20892

Joseph Avruch
Howard Hughes Medical Institute
  Laboratories
Medical Services and Diabetes Unit
Massachusetts General Hospital
Department of Medicine
Harvard Medical School
Boston, Massachusetts 02114

S. Bala-Mohan
Deutches Wollforschungsinstitut an der
  Technischen
Hochschule Aachen
D-51 Aachen, FRG

C. Behrendt
Deutches Wollforschungsinstitut an der
  Technischen
Hochschule Aachen
D-51 Aachen, FRG

John J. M. Bergeron
Departments of Medicine and Anatomy
McGill University and the Royal
  Victoria Hospital
Montreal, Quebec H3A 1A1, Canada

Richard N. Bergman
Department of Physiology and
  Biophysics
USC Medical School
Los Angeles, California 90003

Michel Bernier
Department of Biological Chemistry
The Johns Hopkins University School of
  Medicine
Baltimore, Maryland 21205

Morris J. Birnbaum
Program of Molecular Biology
Memorial Sloan-Kettering Cancer
  Center
New York, New York 10021

Marianne Böni-Schnetzler
Department of Biochemistry
Boston University School of Medicine
Boston, Massachusetts 02118

Dietrich Brandenberg
Deutches Wollforschungsinstitut an der
  Technischen
Hochschule Aachen
D-51 Aachen, FRG

Roger W. Brownsey
Department of Biochemistry
University of British Columbia
Vancouver, British Columbia
  V6T 1W5, Canada

M. Casaretto
Deutches Wollforschungsinstitut an der
  Technischen
Hochschule Aachen
D-51 Aachen, FRG

Elaine Collier
Diabetes Branch
National Institute of Diabetes and
  Digestive and Kidney Diseases
National Institutes of Health
Bethesda, Maryland 20892

Richard Comi
Diabetes Branch
National Institute of Diabetes and
*   Digestive and Kidney Diseases*
National Institutes of Health
Bethesda, Maryland 20892

Samuel W. Cushman
Experimental Diabetes, Metabolism
*   and Nutrition*
MCNEB, National Institute of Diabetes
*   and Digestive and Kidney Diseases*
National Institutes of Health
Bethesda, Maryland 20892

C. Diaconescu
Deutches Wollforschungsinstitut an der
*   Technischen*
Hochschule Aachen
D-51 Aachen, FRG

S. DiPaolo
Experimental Diabetes, Metabolism
*   and Nutrition*
MCNEB, National Institute of Diabetes
*   and Digestive and Kidney Diseases*
National Institutes of Health
Bethesda, Maryland 20892

Yosuke Ebina
Hormone Research Institute
University of California
San Francisco, California 94143-0534

Leland Ellis
Hormone Research Institute
University of California
San Francisco, California 94143-0534

Louise Enns
Department of Medicine
University of Alberta
Edmonton, Alberta T6G 2G3, Canada

I. George Fantus
Polypeptide Hormone Laboratory
Strathcona Medical Building
McGill University
Montreal, Quebec H3A 2B2, Canada

Jose Goldman
Henry Ford Hospital
Detroit, Michigan 48202

Phillip Gorden
Diabetes Branch
National Institute of Diabetes and
*   Digestive and Kidney Diseases*
National Institutes of Health
Bethesda, Maryland 20892

H. Joseph Goren
Department of Medical Biochemistry
University of Calgary
Calgary, Alberta T2N 4N1, Canada

J. Ryan Gunsalus
Howard Hughes Medical Institute
*   Laboratories*
Medical Services and Diabetes Unit
Massachusetts General Hospital
Department of Medicine
Harvard Medical School
Boston, Massachusetts 02114

Howard C. Haspel
Program of Molecular Biology
Memorial Sloan-Kettering Cancer
*   Center*
New York, New York 10021

David Hirshfield
Howard Hughes Medical Institute
*   Laboratories*
Medical Services and Diabetes Unit
Massachusetts General Hospital
Department of Medicine
Harvard Medical School
Boston, Massachusetts 02114

Charles H. Hollenberg
Banting and Best Diabetes Center
University of Toronto
3CCRW845, Toronto General Hospital
Toronto, Ontario M5G 2C4, Canada

Morley D. Hollenberg
Endocrine Research Group
Department of Pharmacology and
*   Therapeutics*
University of Calgary
Faculty of Medicine
Calgary, Alberta T2N 4N1, Canada

Leonard Jarett
Department of Pathology and
Laboratory Medicine
University of Pennsylvania School of
Medicine
Philadelphia, Pennsylvania 19104

Hans G. Joost
Institute for Pharmacology and
Toxicology
AM Pfingstanger 49
D-3400 Göttingen, FRG

C. Ronald Kahn
Research Division
Joslin Diabetes Center
Department of Medicine
Harvard Medical School
Boston, Massachusetts 02215

Masood N. Khan
Departments of Medicine and Anatomy
McGill University and the Royal
Victoria Hospital
Montreal, Quebec H3A 1A1, Canada

Victoria P. Knutson
Department of Pharmacology
The University of Texas Health
Sciences Center at Houston Medical
School
Houston, Texas 77225

Don M. Laird
Department of Biological Chemistry
The Johns Hopkins University School of
Medicine
Baltimore, Maryland 21205

M. Daniel Lane
Department of Biological Chemistry
The Johns Hopkins University School of
Medicine
Baltimore, Maryland 21205

David C. W. Lau
Department of Medicine
University of Calgary
Calgary, Alberta T2N 4N1, Canada

Sushanta Mallick
Department of Biochemistry
University of North Texas
Denton, Texas 76202

Ruthann A. Masaracchia
Department of Biochemistry
University of North Texas
Denton, Texas 76202

David Morgan
Hormone Research Institute
University of California
San Francisco, California 94143-0534

Brian D. Morrison
Department of Physiology and
Biophysics
The University of Iowa
Iowa City, Iowa 52242

M. L. Moule
Banting and Best Department of
Medical Research
University of Toronto
Toronto, Ontario M5G 1L6, Canada

Alice L-F. Mui
Department of Biochemistry
University of British Columbia
Vancouver, British Columbia V6T 1W5,
Canada

Fern E. Murdoch
Department of Biochemistry
University of North Texas
Denton, Texas 76202

Mary Jo O'Sullivan
Departments of Medicine, Pediatrics
and Obstetrics and Gynecology
University of Miami
Miami, Florida 33101

Jeffrey E. Pessin
Department of Physiology and
Biophysics
The University of Iowa
Iowa City, Iowa 52242

M. L. Phillips
Banting and Best Department of
 Medical Research
University of Toronto
Toronto, Ontario M5G 1L6, Canada

Paul F. Pilch
Department of Biochemistry
Boston University School of Medicine
Boston, Massachusetts 02118

Barry I. Posner
Departments of Medicine and Anatomy
McGill University and the Royal
 Victoria Hospital
Montreal, Quebec H3A 1A1, Canada

Katherine A. Quayle
Department of Biochemistry
University of British Columbia
Vancouver, British Columbia V6T 1W5,
Canada

S. Sethu K. Reddy
Research Division
Joslin Diabetes Center
Department of Medicine
Harvard Medical School
Boston, Massachusetts 02215

Ora M. Rosen
Program of Molecular Biology
Memorial Sloan-Kettering Cancer
 Center
New York, New York 10021

Richard A. Roth
Department of Pharmacology
Stanford University
Stanford, California 94305

Dominique Rouiller
Diabetes Branch
National Institute of Diabetes and
 Digestive and Kidney Diseases
National Institutes of Health
Bethesda, Maryland 20892

William J. Rutter
Hormone Research Institute
University of California
San Francisco, California 94143-0534

Edmond A. Ryan
Department of Medicine
University of Alberta
Edmonton, Alberta T6G 2G3, Canada

Benjamin A. Rybicki
Henry Ford Hospital
Detroit, Michigan 48202

Steven Shoelson
Research Division
Joslin Diabetes Center
Department of Medicine
Harvard Medical School
Boston, Massachusetts 02215

Ian A. Simpson
Experimental Diabetes, Metabolism
 and Nutrition
MCNEB, National Institute of Diabetes
 and Digestive and Kidney Diseases
National Institutes of Health
Bethesda, Maryland 20892

Jay S. Skyler
Departments of Medicine, Pediatrics
 and Obstetrics and Gynecology
University of Miami
Miami, Florida 33101

M. Spoden
Deutches Wollforschungsinstitut an der
 Technischen
Hochschule Aachen
D-51 Aachen, FRG

Laurel J. Sweet
Department of Cellular and
 Developmental Biology
Harvard University
Cambridge, Massachusetts 02138

Simeon I. Taylor
Diabetes Branch
National Institute of Diabetes and
 Digestive and Kidney Diseases
National Institutes of Health
Bethesda, Maryland 20892

Hans E. Tornqvist
Department of Pediatrics
University Hospital
University of Lund
S-221 85 Lund, Sweden

M. van de Locht-Blasberg
Deutches Wollforschungsinstitut an der
  Technischen
Hochschule Aachen
D-51 Aachen, FRG

Gerald van de Werve
Laboratoire d'Endocrinologie
  Metabolique
Departement de Nutrition
Universite de Montreal
Montreal, Quebec H3T 1A8, Canada

Lu-Hai Wang
Rockefeller University
New York, New York 10021

Stephen Waugh
Department of Biochemistry
Boston University School of Medicine
Boston, Massachusetts 02118

Teresa M. Weber
Experimental Diabetes, Metabolism
  and Nutrition
MCNEB, National Institute of Diabetes
  and Digestive and Kidney Diseases
National Institutes of Health
Bethesda, Maryland 20892

F. Wedekind
Deutches Wollforschungsinstitut an der
  Technischen
Hochschule Aachen
D-51 Aachen, FRG

Morris F. White
Research Division
Joslin Diabetes Center
Department of Medicine
Harvard Medical School
Boston, Massachusetts 02215

Cecil C. Yip
Banting and Best Department of
  Medical Research
University of Toronto
Toronto, Ontario M5G 1L6, Canada

Kenneth Zierler
Department of Medicine
The Johns Hopkins University School of
  Medicine
Baltimore, Maryland 21205

Insulin Action and Diabetes,
edited by H. Joseph Goren et al.
Raven Press. New York © 1988.

MEMBRANE LINKED INSULIN RECEPTOR TYROSINE KINASE STIMULATES THE INSULIN SPECIFIC RESPONSE

William J. Rutter, David Morgan, Yosuke Ebina,
Lu-Hai Wang[1], Richard Roth[2], and Leland Ellis

Hormone Research Institute, University of California,
San Francisco, CA 94143-0534, [1]Rockefeller University,
New York, N.Y. 10021; [2]Department of Pharmacology,
Stanford University, Stanford, CA 94305

All peptide hormones interact with receptors on the cell surface to engender a specific physiological response. Coincidently, the hormone is internalized and at least in part degraded in the lysosomes. It is possible that the internalized hormone, or its breakdown products, participates in the intracellular response. Alternatively, the interaction of the ligand with the receptor may initiate a regulatory cascade of intracellular reactions that are driven by the receptor and independent of ligand. If this is true, how does the binding of ligand activate the receptor mediated chain of reactions?

We have used the insulin receptor as a paradigm to study the mechanism of action of the peptide hormone receptors. Early studies revealed that the insulin receptor is a heterotetramer comprised of two subunits, α and β, that are derived from a common precursor (2,12). We (3) as well as Ullrich et al (20) have isolated and characterized the human insulin receptor (hIR) cDNA. The sequence of this cDNA revealed the amino acid sequence, and the structural domains of the molecule (Fig. 1). The hIR precursor contains 1355 (3) (or 1343 (20)) amino acids and is ~154,000 (or ~152,000) kd (exclusive of glycosylation); it comprises the α-subunit (N-terminal) and the β-subunit (C-terminal) regions linked by a readily identifiable processing site (four basic amino acids in series). The α-subunit region is preceded by a 27 residue N-terminal signal peptide, and a distinctive cysteine-rich region which we call the cross-linking domain to reflect the ability of cysteine residues to form intra- and intermolecular bonds (3). The β-subunit contains the single transmembrane domain (20 hydrophobic amino acids) and a cytoplasmic region containing a tyrosine kinase (PTK) domain including the putative ATP binding site and tyrosine phosphorylation sites. This tyrosine kinase moiety is structurally related to other tyrosine kinases including the transforming

1

proteins encoded by oncogenes and those in certain transmembrane receptors (EGF (19), PDGF (22), IGFI (21), CSF-I (14), etc). At the C-terminus of the molecule is a region, the "insulin-specific tail", which is rich in hydrophilic and charged residues including many serine, threonine and tyrosine residues that could be sites of phosphorylation. Distinct C-terminal tails also exist in the other receptors. The structural relationship between the insulin and EGF receptors is significant because of their similar functional roles. While the insulin receptor is a heterotetramer α2β2, the EGF receptor exists as a single subunit under most circumstances (see later). Aside from the similarity in the general organization (signal peptide, cross-linking domain, transmembrane domain, tyrosine kinase and EGF or insulin-specific tail) there is no obvious relationship at the level of amino acid sequence, except in the organization of cysteine residues in the cysteine-rich domain, and in the sequence similarity in the tyrosine kinase region (3). In contrast, the IGF-I receptor sequence (21; J. Edman & W. Rutter, unpublished) is quite similar to the insulin receptor and particularly strong in the tyrosine kinase domain (84%), in regions surrounding the cross-linking domain (67%, 64%), and in the intracellular domain between the PTK and the transmembrane domains (61%); the remaining portions have low similarity (41-48%). Thus, the closely related insulin and IGF-I receptors appear to have arisen evolutionarily from a common precursor. On the other hand the evolution of the EGF receptor is less clear; it may have evolved via the recruitment of single domains rather than by strictly linear derivation from a common ancestor.

The search for the biological role of the receptors naturally centers on the tyrosine kinase moiety, the most plausible active component of the intracellular domain. Ligand binding stimulates tyrosine kinase activity in most receptors of the tyrosine kinase family (11). In the case of the IR, insulin binding stimulates dramatically the activity of the tyrosine kinase (2,12) (Fig. 1). This stimulation could be related to internalization and the representation of the receptor of the cell surface since this process also is stimulated by ligand binding. On the other hand, the tyrosine kinase could be the direct actor in the specific physiological response. In this case, the physiological specificity of the response is presumably due to an array of interacting molecules with the specificity resulting from the intrinsic specificity of the PTK to phosphorylate a selected subset of possible proteins, or to physical contiguity of the molecules. What is the structural essence of the functional differences between the oncogenic tyrosine kinases and the more limited and directed activities of the receptor tyrosine kinases? Save for the IGF-I receptor (21), the insulin receptor is most closely related to the v-ros oncogene tyrosine kinase (14) which, in the context of a chicken retrovirus, produces sarcomas. v-ros, like pp60src (7,18) and v-erbB (21), is linked to the membrane and has few extracellular sequences. Thus it, like other oncogenic tyrosine kinases, has no ligand

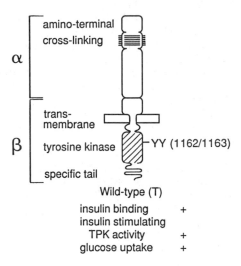

FIG. 1. The structural domains of the insulin receptor and the generation of the insulin response in cells.

binding site and lacks a C-terminal domain analogous to the hormone-specific tail. Does the tail modify the function of the tyrosine kinase?

The sequence similarities between the various tyrosine kinases are not high. Each contains an ATP binding site consisting of a consensus sequence, Gly-X-Gly-X-X-Gly (11), about 10 bases upstream from a presumably critical lysine residue. The possible sites of phosphorylation include tyrosines in the vicinity of the ATP binding domain, others within the central region of the kinase itself, including a conserved tyrosine that is a phosphorylation site in most tyrosine kinases, and tyrosine residues in the tail region.

In order to elucidate the functions of the various domains of the receptor we have selectively mutated the cDNA so that the resultant receptor is modified in the regions of interest (7). Either the receptor is truncated to eliminate certain portions of the molecule or specifically mutated at a particular amino acid or sequence by site-directed mutagenesis. The mutated cDNA is then expressed under transcriptional control of the SV40 early promoter in a specifically designed expression plasmid in Chinese hamster ovary (CHO) cells (4,6). Co-transfection with a plasmid carrying the bacterial gene for neomycin resistance allows the isolation of stably transformed CHO cells containing the native or mutant hIR sequences. Selection for cells expressing high levels of hIR is then conveniently done using fluorescence-activated cell sorting (FACS). Human receptors can be distinguished from the endogenous hamster receptors via monoclonal antibodies specific for the hIR protein (4). hIR, expressed in this manner, is functional (4); it exhibits normal insulin binding and insulin stimulated phosphorylation of the β-subunit (Fig. 1). Furthermore, it mediates insulin-activated uptake of 2-deoxyglucose (3). Overexpression of the hIR 10-fold compared to the endogenous hamster receptors results in a 10-20 fold shift in the insulin sensitivity of the cells, half-maximal stimulation of the uptake of insulin occurs at 10^{-11} to 10^{-12}M (10x hIR overexpression) instead of 10^{-9} to 10^{-10}M (normal CHO cells) insulin concentration! This is understandable qualitatively since the amount of ligand required to saturate an internal response decreases with an increased number of receptors on the cell surface. However, the number of bound insulin molecules required to achieve an insulin-specific response decreases from 500-1000 (in normal CHO cells) to 50-100 receptors (10x hIR in CHO cells)! The receptors act more efficiently in the cells with larger number of receptors on the cell surface. Thus the signal provided by the binding of an insulin molecule is somehow amplified by the proximity of other receptors. These effects can be eliminated by adding hIR-specific monoclonal antibodies; thus they are specifically associated with the human receptor. One explanation for this phenomenon is that the ligand binding to one receptor is communicated to other receptors in the vicinity. In further experiments using mutant receptors, cells expressing the levels of the receptors were selected by FACS using monoclonal antibodies labeled with a fluorescent probe (6,7). In this manner, cells were obtained with fifty to several hundred times higher mutant receptor concentrations, compared to the endogenous receptor concentrations. The physiological activity of the receptors (insulin binding, insulin stimulated tyrosine kinase activity) was measured and the presence and conformation of the various receptor domains were tested with the monoclonal antibodies of Roth (17).

The results of the series of mutation experiments suggest that various domains of the insulin receptor assume the appropriate conformation and function independently of each other. Thus truncation experiments in which portions of the molecule are eliminated, can be used to discern the function of the domains.

INSULIN RECEPTORS REQUIRE A FUNCTIONAL TYROSINE KINASE CYTOPLASMIC DOMAIN FOR BIOLOGICAL FUNCTION

A number of different experiments demonstrate that a mutant hIR in which the tyrosine kinase domain is either lost or crippled, can bind insulin normally but does not stimulate glucose uptake. Thus tyrosine kinase activity and a functional cytoplasmic domain is required to generate the insulin specific response; insulin uptake in the cell is not sufficient. If the insulin specific tail is removed, this somehow destabilizes the entire intracellular domain such that the molecule is terminated (processed?) close to the transmembrane domain. This molecule

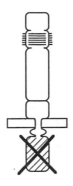

T-t

insulin binding	+
insulin stimulating	
TPK activity	-
glucose uptake	-

FIG. 2. The insulin response requires an intracellular domain. The carboxyterminal 112 residues (including the tail) are required for de novo folding of a functional PTK domain; elimination of these residues results in less of the intracellular domain. The insulin binding and internalization is normal but the biological response is lost.

binds insulin (6), and transports it into the cell normally (Berhanu et al., unpublished), but has no effect on glucose uptake (Fig. 2).

Similarly, replacement of the C-terminal domain with the intracellular domains of the bacterial chemotactic receptor yields a chimera which binds insulin normally, but does not stimulate glucose uptake (8). Finally, replacement of the lysine residue (supposedly functioning in the ATP binding site) with arginine, methionine, or alanine residues also results in normal insulin binding, but this receptor mutant does not stimulate glucose uptake (5). In this instance the tyrosine kinase activity is also eliminated, confirming the crucial role of this lysine in tyrosine kinase function, presumably in the binding of ATP.

PHOSPHORYLATION OF THE TYROSINE KINASE IS A REQUISITE FOR THE INSULIN-SPECIFIC RESPONSE

To test whether insulin-stimulated phosphorylation of the tyrosine kinase moiety is important in the physiological response, we replaced with phenylalanine one or both of the tyrosines at the conserved central phosphorylation site (position 1162/1163) of the tyrosine kinase (6) (Fig. 3). These isomorphic replacements did not prevent phosphorylation on other tyrosines and serines in the molecule but they partially compromised (1 tyrosine → phenylalanine) or nearly eliminated (2

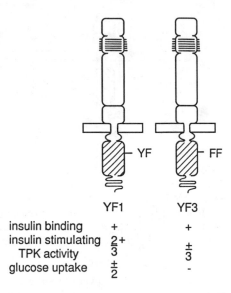

insulin binding	+	+
insulin stimulating TPK activity	$\frac{2}{3}$+	$\pm\frac{1}{3}$
glucose uptake	$\pm\frac{1}{2}$	-

FIG. 3. Phosphorylation on tyrosine residues (1162/1163) is required for physiological response. Mutation to phenylalanine permits phosphorylation at other sites, but the insulin response is severely compromised.

tyrosines → 2 phenylalanines) the insulin stimulation of glucose uptake. Thus tyrosine phosphorylation appears to be required for the insulin specific response, and this site is somehow particularly significant. Other sites of phosphorylation are known; these may complement or replace phosphorylation at this site in the physiological response. This experimental result lends persuasive support to the hypothesis that insulin stimulated phosphorylation of the tyrosine kinase is the basis of receptor-mediated cell functions.

A TRUNCATED INSULIN RECEPTOR COMPRISED OF A MEMBRANE-LINKED INTRACELLULAR DOMAIN IS FULLY FUNCTIONAL IN GENERATING A PHYSIOLOGICAL RESPONSE

Reconstruction of the hIR cDNA such that the α-subunit is virtually eliminated by linking the signal peptide directly to the extracellular portion of the β-subunit results in the expression of a molecular analogue of the oncogenic tyrosine kinase of v-ros (Fig. 4) (9). Not surprisingly this molecule does not bind to insulin. However, it displays very high constitutive levels of tyrosine kinase activity, about the same level of activity observed when the insulin is bound to the native receptor! Remarkably, the glucose uptake of the cells expressing SpBam is constitutively high. Further, replacement with phenylalanine of the two tyrosines 1162/1163 at the phosphorylation site eliminates this high glucose uptake (Fig. 4). Thus the

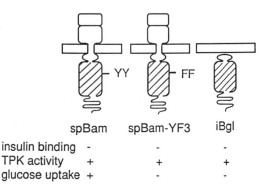

	spBam	spBam-YF3	iBgl
insulin binding	-	-	-
TPK activity	+	+	+
glucose uptake	+	-	-

FIG. 4. The elimination of ligand binding domain confers constitutive function. Truncation of the α-subunit increases PTK activity, and stimulates glucose uptake, provided that the extracellular domain is bound to the membrane. Overexpression of the cytoplasmic PTK as in iBgl results in high levels of PTK activity, but no insulin-specific response.

stimulation of glucose uptake is mediated by the tyrosine kinase in the absence of the hormone. It appears that the activity of the tyrosine kinase is somehow repressed in the presence of the extracellular domain. Ligand binding relieves the repression and the intrinsic activity of the tyrosine kinase then produces the biological response. This result clarifies the interpretation of earlier experimental results involving certain monoclonal antibodies to the insulin receptor which exert an insulin like effect. They must bind to the insulin receptor in a way that eliminates the inhibitory influence of the extracellular domain. (This does not imply that they must have an insulin-like configuration at the binding site.)

The observations are also consistent with the finding that glucose uptake can be stimulated by treatment of cells with proteolytic enzymes such as trypsin. Conceivably, the proteolytic enzymes remove or modify the extracellular domain and thus activate the intracellular tyrosine kinase.

If the receptor cDNA coding sequences for the extracellular domain and the transmembrane domain are removed, the cytoplasmic region of the hIR can be expressed in cells and the tyrosine kinase is fully active in the cytoplasm (9). However, even when overexpressed more than 100 times relative to the endogenous IR, this molecule does not activate glucose uptake (Fig. 4). Thus it seems for this function, the tyrosine kinase must be displayed in the context of the membrane. Apparently the cytoplasmic tyrosine kinase molecules do not reach the physiological site in sufficient quantity to effectuate the insulin-specific response on glucose uptake.

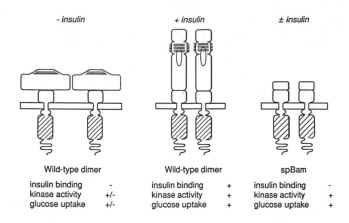

FIG. 5. Model of the role of the extracellular domain and ligand binding in generating the specific physiological response. In this hypothesis, the intrinsic activity of the PTK is compromised by the structure of the extracellular domain (here indicated as the conformation of the α-subunit). This results in the inability to transphosphorylate and hence acti- vate the neighboring PTK subunit. The binding of the ligand relieves this inhibition by altering the configuration.

INTERSUBUNIT TRANSPHORYLATION -- A MODEL FOR TRANSMEMBRANE SIGNALLING

Ligand activation of tyrosine kinase in peptide hormone receptors is a reflection of transmembrane signalling (7). To explain this phenomenon we hypothesize that the "phosphoryla- tion" associated with activation process is really transphos- phorylation between the adjacent tyrosine kinase moieties of the dimeric structures (Fig. 5). As is the case with other enzymatic interactions, intermolecular rather than intramolecular reac- tions predominate. We assume that the extracellular domain in the absence of ligand assumes a configuration or interacts with other components of the membrane (integral proteins having cysteine rich domains?) so that transphosphorylation is inhi- bited and that ligand binding restores the functional inter- active state of the tyrosine kinases. This hypothesis is consis- tent with several of our experimental observations. 1) Expres- sion of compromised (mutated) insulin receptors inhibits the effectiveness of endogenous CHO receptors in stimulating glucose uptake. We presume that dimers are formed in which transphos- phorylation is either inhibited or blocked (Fig. 6). 2) Mem- brane-linked truncated receptors are fully functional, pre- sumably because of the absence of the constraints of the extra- cellular domain (7). 3) The increased efficiency of ligand activation by overexpression of receptors on the cell surface (3) can be explained. If heterotetramers can form clusters, then

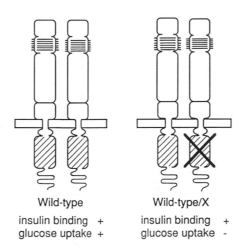

Wild-type   Wild-type/X

insulin binding +   insulin binding   +
glucose uptake +   glucose uptake   -

FIG. 6. Dimers and multimers required for IR function. If transphosphorylation of PTK subunits is involved in activation, then dimers formed with an inactive subunit will inhibit PTK activity.

ligand binding may result in an activation of multiple hetero-tetramers based on physical contiguity of the tyrosine kinases. This hypothesis is also consistent with results of others who show that the functional heterotetramer is required for activation of tyrosine kinase but once activated, the α,β heterodimer is sufficient (1,17,18). In support of this view other single chain receptors such as EGF apparently form dimers during activation of the receptor. Transmembrane signalling therefore may be the result of specific intermolecular communication.

REPLACEMENT OF THE INSULIN RECEPTOR TYROSINE KINASE WITH THE
V-ROS TYROSINE KINASE RESULTS IN LIGAND-MEDIATED TRANSMEMBRANE
SIGNALLING BUT NO INSULIN-SPECIFIC RESPONSE

In order to test whether the intrinsic specificity of the tyrosine kinase is required for the hormone specific response, we replaced the tyrosine kinase domain of the IR with the tyrosine kinase domain of the oncogene, v-ros (10). When expressed, the resultant IR/v-ros is displayed normally on the cell membrane. Interaction with insulin stimulates v-ros tyrosine kinase activity (although to a lower degree than the native tyrosine kinase). In spite of this, when the IR/v-ros is over-expressed in CHO cells there is no stimulation of the endogenous glucose uptake in the presence of insulin. Moreover, the stimulation of thymidine uptake ordinarily observed with the v-ros

containing chicken retrovirus is also not observed in the
IR/v-ros. Apparently the v-ros tyrosine kinase, when present
within the context of the insulin receptor, no longer behaves as
an oncogene. In addition, the IR-v-ros cannot replace the normal
insulin receptor tyrosine kinase. These results suggest that the
substrate specificity of the tyrosine kinase is an important
component of the hormone specific response. This result is
consistent with the diversity of structures represented in
members of the tyrosine kinase family.

UNREGULATED EXPRESSION OF A MEMBRANE-LINKED INSULIN RECEPTOR TYROSINE KINASE TRANSFORMS CELLS

The biological activity of the truncated, membrane-linked
insulin receptor tyrosine kinase was tested by Wang et al. (23)
by placing it under the control of the LTR promoter in a pseudo
retrovirus vector. Expression of this insulin receptor tyrosine
kinase in chicken embryo fibroblasts results in cell transformation as measured by growth in soft agar, altered cell mor-
phology, and the development of distinctive foci. On the other
hand, this recombinant IR-containing retrovirus did not produce
tumors in chickens. However, rapidly growing variants of these
cells exhibited more distorted growth patterns, distinctive foci
in culture and tumors in animals. Thus it appears that unregu-
lated and continuous production of high levels of the insulin

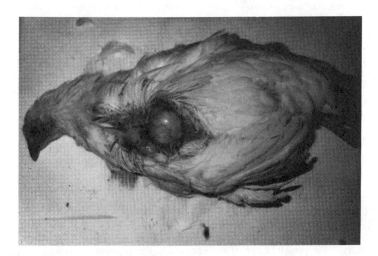

FIG. 7. Tumors formed from rapidly growing variant cell VR
derived by transforming chicken embryo fibroblasts with a
retrovirus vector, pUIR, in which the protein tyrosine kinase-
containing region of the hIR is fused at its 5' end to part of
the viral gag portion of the v-ros under transcriptional control
of the LTR (23).

receptor kinase exerts an abnormal effect on growth. Further, modifications in tyrosine kinase structure somehow alter the activity or specificity of the tyrosine kinase such that it is able to activate factors limiting cell proliferation. These tyrosine kinase mutants are then selected for because they activate cell proliferation. These results are consistent with the view that the physiological specificity of the receptor tyrosine kinases is dependent on its molecular context, on its intrinsic specificity and on the regulation of its expression. Thus, oncogenicity may result from mutations in the extracellular domain that relieve the suppression of the tyrosine kinase activity of the receptor and/or mutations in the tyrosine kinase moiety to influence its activity or specificity.

REFERENCES

1. Boni-Schnetzler, M., Rubin, J.B., and Pilch, P.F., (1986): J. Biol. Chem.. 261:15281-15287.
2. Czech, M.P. (1985): Ann. Rev. Physiol., 47:357-381.
3. Ebina, Y., Ellis, L., Jarnagin, K., Edery, M., Graf, L., Clauser, E., Ou, J., Masiarz, F., Roth, R.A., and Rutter, W.J. (1985): Cell, 41:747-758.
4. Ebina, Y., Edery, M., Ellis, L., Standring, D., Beaudoin, J., Roth, R.A., and Rutter, W.J., (1985): Proc. Nat. Acad. Sci. USA, 82:8014-8018.
5. Ebina, Y., Araki, E., Taira, M., Shimada, F., Mori, M., Craik, C.S., Siddle, K., Pierce, S.B., Roth, R.A., and Rutter, W.J., (1987): Proc. Nat. Acad. Sci. USA, 84: 704-708.
6. Ellis, L., Clauser, E., Morgan, D.O., Edery, M., Roth, R.A., and Rutter, W.J. (1986): Cell, 45:721-732.
7. Ellis, L., Morgan, D.O., Clauser, E., Edery, M., Jong, S.-M., Wang, L.-H., Roth, R.A., and Rutter, W.J., (1986): Cold Spring Harbor Symp. Quant. Biol., 51:773-784.
8. Ellis, L., Morgan, D.O., Koshland, D.E., Jr., Clauser, E., Moe, G.R., Bollag, G., Roth, R.A., and Rutter, W.J., (1986): Proc. Nat. Acad. Sci. USA, 83:8137-8141.
9. Ellis, L., Morgan, D.O., Clauser, E., Roth, R.A., and Rutter, W.J., (1987): Mol. Endocrinol., 1:15-24.
10. Ellis, L., Morgan, D.O., Jong, S.-M., Wang, L.-H., Roth, R.A., and Rutter, W.J., (1987): Proc. Nat. Acad. Sci. USA, 84:5101-5105.
11. Hunter, T. and Cooper, J.A. (1985): Ann. Rev. Biochem., 54:897-930.
12. Kahn, C.R. 1985. Ann. Rev. Med., 36:429-451.
13. Morgan, D.O., and Roth, R.A., (1986): Biochemistry, 25: 1364-1371.
14. Neckameyer, W.S., and Wang, L.-H., (1985): J. Virol., 53: 879-884.
15. Pessin, J.E., Sweet, L.J., and Morrison, B.D., this volume.
16. Pilch, P., et al., this volume.

17. Roth, R.A., Cassell, D.J., Wong, K.Y., Maddux, B.A., and Goldfine, I.D. (1982). Proc. Nat. Acad. Sci. USA, 79:7312.
18. Smart, J.E., Oppermann, H., Czernilofsky, A.P., Purchio, A.F., Erikson, R.L., and Bishop, J.M., (1981): Proc. Nat. Acad. Sci. USA, 78:6013.
19. Ullrich, A., Coussens, L., Hayflick, J.S., Dull, T.J., Gray, H., Lee, J., Yarden, Y., Libermann, T.A., Schlessinger, J., Downward, J., Mayes, E.L.V., Whittle, N., Waterfield, M.D., and Seeburg, P.H., (1984): Nature, 309: 418-425.
20. Ullrich, A., Bell, J.R., Chen, E.Y., Herrera, R., Petruzelli, L.M., Dull, T.J., Gray, A., Coussens, L., Liao, Y.-C., Tsubokawa, M., Mason, A., Seeburg, P.H., Grunfeld, C., Rosen, O.M., and Ramachandran, J., (1985): Nature, 313:756-761.
21. Ullrich, A., Gray, A., Tam, A.W., Yang-Feng, T., Tsubokawa, M., Collins, C., Henzel, W., Le Bon, T., Kathuria, S., Chen, E., Jacobs, S., Francke, U., Ramachandran, J., and Fujita-Yamaguchi, Y., (1986): EMBO J., 5:2503-2512.
22. Yarden, Y., Escobedo, J.A., Kuang, W.J., Yang-Feng, T.L., Daniel, T.O., Tremble, P.M., Chen, E.Y., Ando, M.E., Harkins, R.N., Francke, U., Fried, V.A., Ullrich, A., and Williams, L.T., (1986): Nature, 323:226-232.
23. Wang, L.-H., Lin, B., Jong, S.-M., Dixon, D., Ellis, L., Roth, R.A., and Rutter, W.J., (1987): Proc. Nat. Acad. Sci. USA, 84:5725-5729.

Insulin Action and Diabetes,
edited by H. Joseph Goren et al.
Raven Press, New York © 1988.

SEMISYNTHETIC AND PHOTOREACTIVE ANALOGUES

FOR STUDIES OF INSULIN RECEPTOR AND INSULIN ACTION

D. Brandenburg, D. Ambrosius, S. Bala-Mohan,
C. Behrendt, M. Casaretto, C. Diaconescu, M. Spoden,
M. van de Löcht-Blasberg, F. Wedekind

Deutsches Wollforschungsinstitut an der Technischen
Hochschule Aachen, D-51 Aachen, Fed. Rep. Germany

INTRODUCTION

Elucidating the still largely unknown molecular mechanism of insulin action (22,30) is a complex, which requires approaches from different directions and at different levels. Insulin chemistry provides a basis for a variety of studies and for the development of variants exhibiting improved therapeutic properties. Although the hormone is a polyfunctional macromolecule (Figures 1,2), methods for rather sophisticated chemistry could be developed, allowing the preparation of numerous analogues and derivatives for structure-function studies under reversible conditions (9,39,49). Moreover, they also led to a series of derivatives for irreversible anchoring to the receptor (43,57).

The purpose of this paper is to outline recent developments, employing examples from our Laboratory and collaborative studies. First, various synthetic and semisynthetic approaches as well as some structure-function relationships will be presented. The work on shortened insulin amides is discussed in more detail. Second, results from photo-affinity labelling experiments of the insulin receptor will be summarized, followed by a description of the design and the preparation of new photo-reactive insulins.

13

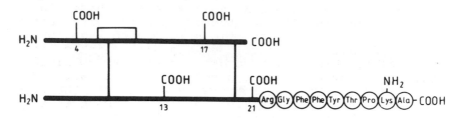

FIG.1. Simplified primary structure of insulin, showing
the 3 amino groups (N-terminal, and B29-lysine), the 6
carboxyl groups (2 C-terminal, 4 glutamic acids), and
the C-terminal amino acids of the B-chain.

INSULIN ANALOGUES

Insulins with Various Structural Alteration

Total synthesis
Based on our previous work (8), several A- and B-
chains have been built up by total synthesis in
solution, using fragment condensation, and have subsequently been combined with their natural counter chain.
A-chains with mono and diiodo tyrosine in position 19
(55), chicken A-chain (56), and an A-chain with a C-
terminal extension by the IGF I octapeptide sequence
63-70 (31) have been obtained. B-chains were altered by
replacing B17-leucine by D-Leu or Nle (32), or 22-Arg
by D-Arg (33). Combination yields can be markedly
increased by recycling material with incorrectly paired
cystine disulfide bonds (46).

Semisynthesis and chemical modification.
Citraconyl insulins have been prepared as partially
protected intermediates and for stucture-function
studies (37). Semisynthesis (review: ref. 49) led to a
series of analogues with modified position A1 through
Edman degradation of B1,B29-protected insulin and specific acylations at A2 (52). Removal of the next three
amino acids and re-addition of synthetic tetrapeptides
appeared promising (52), but requires more intense
investigation. Enzyme-assisted semisynthesis was
studied in some detail and led to several analogues
through the addition of tetra- and octapeptides to des-
(B23-B30)-insulin and amino acid derivatives to des-
B30-Ala-insulin (23). B16-Tyrosine could be selectively
exchanged in the isolated B-chain by enzymatic/chemical
techniques (24).

Crosslinking
Intramolecular crosslinking created a new derivative
with D-Ala in positions A1 and B1 (44), while intermolecular joining of diprotected insulins with active
esters of suberic or sebacic acid led to the preparation of all six possible dimers with linked amino
groups (47). Finally, a covalent dimer was obtained by
cooxidation of two semisynthetic insulins with B25-
cysteines (21). It is structurally related to the dimer
formed by association of two insulin monomers in solution or in the crystal (see refs. 5,7).

Structure-function relationships
Cooperative studies with these analogues gave
further information on the relationships between
primary structure, conformation, receptor binding and
biological activities. For example, the hybrid chicken/
human insulin exhibited elevated activity, as expected
(56), while the C-terminal extension of the A-chain
decreased metabolic, but increased growth promoting
activity (31). B22-D-Arg, B17-D-Leu and B17-Nle
analogues showed binding and glucose oxidation values
in adipocytes of 2, about 10 and 20%, respectively,
while DNA synthesis in cultured human fibroblasts was
16, 35 and 100%, compared with insulin (32,33).
    The low activity (9%) of crosslinked insulin is
obviously due to restriction of the flexibility required for binding (44). In vivo, such molecules cause
hypoglycemia in dogs by inhibition of hepatic glucose
production, but not peripheral glucose uptake (12).
    It is noteworthy that covalent insulin dimers gen-
erally exhibit reduced potency in vitro (2% for B29-
B29' to 55% for B1-B29'- dimer), while receptor binding
is up to tenfold (B29-B29'-dimer) higher (47). Stimulation of receptor kinase is correlated to biopotency,
while receptor down-regulation is related to occupancy
(42). Some evidence on the mechanism of insulin receptor interaction and binding stoichiometry has been
derived from comparisons of such dimers with asymmetri-
cal insulin-des(B23-B30)-insulin dimers (51).
    The C-terminus of the B-chain has received parti-
cular attention in our recent and current research.
The finding, that the covalent B25-B25'-dimer is almost
inactive, favours the concept that at least part of the
dimer-forming surface of insulin is directly involved
in contacts with the receptor (21).
    A detailed study of B24- and B25-Leu-insulins did
not confirm literature data indicating antagonism to
insulin (15).

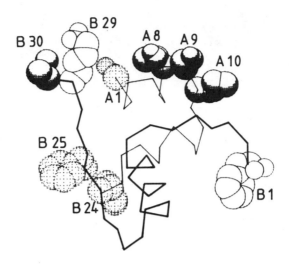

FIG.2. Simplified 3-dimensional structure of insulin
(see refs. 5,7). The main-chains of the A-chain (——)
and the B-chain (▬▬) are represented by their line-
connected C-atoms. Some side-chains are shown in space-
filling representation: Sites where photo reagents were
attached (open), residues thought to participate in
receptor binding (dotted), and those differing in species (human, porcine, bovine) insulins (heavy shading).
Figure prepared with ACAMOD and reproduced from ref. 36
with permission).

C-terminally Shortened Insulin Amides

Semisynthesis
Our interest focused on des-pentapeptide(B26-B30)-
insulin and related molecules. Such analogues are
easily accessible through trypsin-assisted semisynthesis from des-(B23-B30)-insulin and synthetic peptides (20) on the basis of the initial work of Morihara
(see 49) and the systematic studies of Gattner (23,49).
The procedure is outlined in Fig.3. Acid-cleavable
protecting groups are usually used for the preparation
of amides (left), while a combination of alkali-labile
amino protection with acid-labile carboxyl protection
(right) allowed sequential deblocking and intermediate
purification. With 10 - 15 equivalents of peptide,
couplings at pH 6.5 in dimethylformamide/glycerol/water
usually proceed to about 90% within 12 hours at room
temperature. After final ion exchange chromatography on
DE-cellulose at pH 8, most analogues are pure by
approx. 95% according to RP-HPLC . Selected des-(B26-
B30)-insulins are listed in Table I.

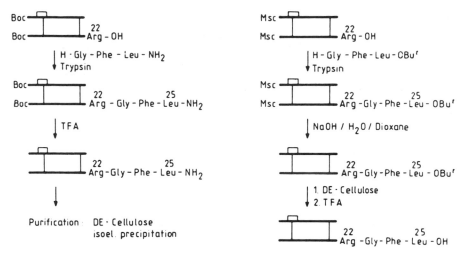

FIG.3. Reaction scheme for the preparation of insulin analogues with shortened C-terminus of the B-chain. Boc = t-butyloxycarbonyl, Msc = methylsulfonylethyloxy-carbonyl, TFA = trifluoro acetic acid (from ref. 19 with permission).

Properties
Des(B26-B30)-insulin. This "parent compound" is monomeric in solution and in the crystal (5). X-ray analysis shows a similar main chain arrangement as 2-zinc insulin . The reduced activity in vitro has been interpreted to indicate that at least some of the lacking residues are essential for binding. There-fore,we were surprised to find that the B25-amide exhi-bited full potency (20). This shows that the shortened molecule contains already all of the structural and dynamic properties required for recognition and binding by the receptor and for exertion of the biological effects. In the presence of a charged carboxylic group in an otherwise hydrophobic environment these are im-paired. These results were confirmed by Nakagawa and Tager (38) and our Chinese colleagues (Zhang, Y.-S., personal communication).

Based on these observations, our studies were exten-ded to replacements which in the intact insulin mole-cule lead to decreased or elevated activity.

B25-Analogues. Independent studies (19,38) have demonstrated that the presence of Leu in position B25 is clearly less detrimental than in the mutant insulin Chicago. Considerable activity inspite of lacking B25-Phe shed some doubt on the absolute importance of the aromatic ring . On the other hand, reduction of potency under obvious retainment of 3-dimensional structure, as evidenced by CD, pointed towards a rather specific role.

TABLE 1. Insulin analogues and photo-reactive
                    derivatives

Modified insulin		% Yield[a]	% Biopot.[b]	Ref.
1. Des-pentapeptide-insulins				
des-(B26-B30)			15 - 35	cf.20
des-(B26-B30), B25-amide		26	105	20
B25-Leu		36	8	19
B25-Leu	, B25-amide	37	18	19
B24-D-Phe	, B25-amide	39	8	11
B25-D-Phe	, B25-amide	52	0.5	11
B25-Trp	, B25-amide	34	54	11
B25-Tyr	, B25-amide	25	228	11
B25-His	, B25-amide	42	313	11
2. Photo-reactive derivatives				
des-(B26-B30)-insulin-B25-Ed-Nap		6	45	3,2
B29,B29'-(Nap-Ahx)$_2$-B1-B1'-		5	2	1,2
azelaoyl-dimer				
B29-(Nap-Lys(Biot))-insulin		31	19	54
Abz-Proinsulin		10	nd	53

[a]Based on insulin. [b]Lipogenesis in isolated rat fat
cells, calculated on a molar basis as ED_{50}(insulin)/
ED_{50}(analogue) x 100. Maximal insulin effect was
achieved in all cases at sufficiently high concentrations. Abbreviations: Abz = 4-azidobenzoyl, Ahx = 6-
aminohexanoyl, Biot = biotinyl, Nap = 2-nitro-4-azido-
phenyl, Ed = $HN-CH_2-CH_2-NH$.

        Its importance was further investigated in a   series
of   experiments   employing   aromatic   replacements (see
Table).   The   dramatic loss of activity with the   D-Phe
analogue   stresses the dependance on   stereospecificity
in this region. A moderate loss of activity with tryp-
tophane   in position B25 is antagonized by the increase
of potency by the hydroxyphenyl side chain of tyrosine,
as found in Aachen (11) and Chicago (38).
        Most   recently it was found by M.   Spoden (ref.11)
that a further increase in potency can be achieved. The
incorporation   of   histidine in position B25 yields   an
analogue which, although shortened by five amino acids,
exhibits threefold insulin activity in vitro.   Inspite
of a wide range of activity CD spectra show no significant structural differences. Thus, the overall conformation of the analogues does not seem to be affected by
the B25 side-chain. It may thus be that the side-chain
of residue B25 interacts with the receptor, but   there
is no direct evidence. A balanced proportion of aromatic and polar character appears to be required for

optimal receptor interaction. Molecular dynamics and computer graphics have shown that the B25-Phe ring is highly flexible. Consequently, it may have a specific dynamic function in building up the hormone-receptor contacts of this region.

Position B24. Finally, we tested the replacement of B24-Phe. It has been reported (34), that in insulin D-Phe leads to enhanced receptor binding (180%) and activity in vitro (140%). With the shortened insulin, such enhancing effects were not observed. Instead, the potency dropped to a value below 10%.

Conclusions
Sequence alterations, which in the intact insulin molecule cause a marked reduction of activity, as well as modifications which enhance potency, are modulated in a sense that they become less pronounced in the shortened analogues. The C-terminal "tail" of the last five amino acids possibly brings about a certain rigidity - which may have negative or positive consequences - while the shorter molecules are more flexible, and the effects are levelled.

PHOTO-REACTIVE INSULINS

Insulins which have been derivatized with light-activatable groups ("photo-insulins") and in most cases additionally labelled with 125-iodine, have proved to be valuable tools in receptor research (reviews: 10, 43, 57). While some information can already be obtained with crude, non-fractionated materials, carefully prepared and characterized photo-insulins with defined substitutions are clearly superior and often indispensable.

Studies under reversible conditions (see above) give only indirect information on the binding surfaces of insulin and its receptor. In contrast, Abz-insulins, introduced by C.C. Yip (57) and also applied by others (e.g.14), and Napa-insulins, developed in our Institute by P. Thamm (see 43), have given direct evidence for the proximity of both N-termini and the B-chain C-terminus (see Figures 1,2) to the receptor surface. Much further information could be obtained, and results with our Napa-insulins are summarized below.

Recent Applications of Napa-insulins

Structural characterization
2-Nitro-4-azidophenylacetyl-insulins (mostly B2-Napa-des-Phe-insulins, but also B29- and occasionally A1-derivatives) have been used for structural characterization of insulin receptors in different cells

(10,16), of rat brown adipose tissue (50), of an insulin producing cell line (RINm5F)(25), and during embryogenesis of rabbits (40). Receptors of brain (26) and of cultured hypothalamic cells (13) have been differentiated against those of normal target tissues. Molecular associations between insulin receptors and major histocompatibility complex class I antigens have been detected (16,17).

On the basis of Ferguson analyses the apparent mass of the α-subunit (M_r ca.130.000) has been corrected to 100.000 (10). Careful tryptic digestion studies of the insulin-receptor complex led J. Neffe to propose a refined model of the binding subunit (see 10).

Fate and activity of the covalent complex
The dynamics of internalization (4) and recycling of insulin-receptor complexes (27) have been studied in adipocytes; properties of nuclear translocation (41), and also processing of insulin (28) and of the receptor have been investigated (29) in isolated hepatocytes.

The persistent lipogenesis, brought about by covalent linking photo-insulins to viable adipocytes (10) has been further investigated with respect to time-course (48) and inhibition by monoclonal anti-insulin antibodies (36).

New Photo-reactive Derivatives

Several new photo-activatable molecules were designed and prepared as specific tools for more detailed studies on receptor structure and function.

Des-(B26-B30)-insulin-B25-(4-Nap-iminoethyleneamide)
The finding, that des-(B26-B30)-insulin amide is fully active and that analogues with replacements in position 25 display very interesting properties, suggested that residue B25 might be in direct contact with the receptor (see above). Therefore, the first insulin derivative bearing a light-sensitive group in a C-terminal position was prepared (2,3).

The peptide (Fig 4.) was obtained by coupling Nap-ethylene diamine to the Boc-tripeptide. It was then condensed with des-(B23-B30)-insulin according to the enzymatic procedure described above. Deblocking and purification gave the desired compound in a high state of purity, as shown by HPLC. Comparison with amides of similar structure, but without nitro and azido functions demonstrated, that these additional groups do not interfere with activity and reversible binding. Thus, the new derivative fulfills the requirements of a probe for this putative binding site.

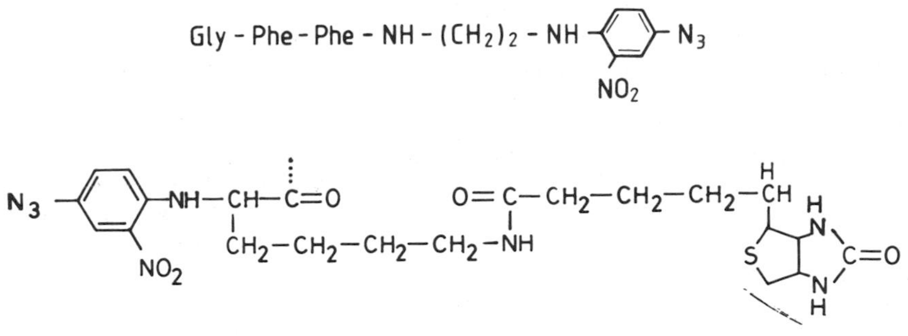

Gly – Phe – Phe – NH – $(CH_2)_2$ – NH –⟨ ⟩– N_3
NO₂ (under ring)

FIG.4. Top: Structure of the tripeptide with a C-terminal photo-reactive substituent (3). Bottom: Structure of the lysine derivative for labelling insulin in position B29 (S. Bala-Mohan, unpubl.)

B29,B29'-Bis(Nap-Ahx)-B1-B1'-azelaoyl-insulin-dimer

Since the insulin receptor is a hetero-tetramer containing two α-subunits, one receptor molecule can principally bind two insulins. So far, the question of binding stoichiometry has not been unequivocally solved. While most authors appear to favour monovalency (e.g.51), others found a ratio of insulin:receptor of 1 (18). It may well be that stoichiometry depends on the state of the receptor, its environment and the experimental conditions (see also 22,30).

In order to study receptor valency, as well as intermolecular relationships between different receptors - for instance in conjunction with receptor aggregation and clustering - we have prepared a dimeric, bivalent photo-insulin (1,2). The structure is outlined in Figure 5.

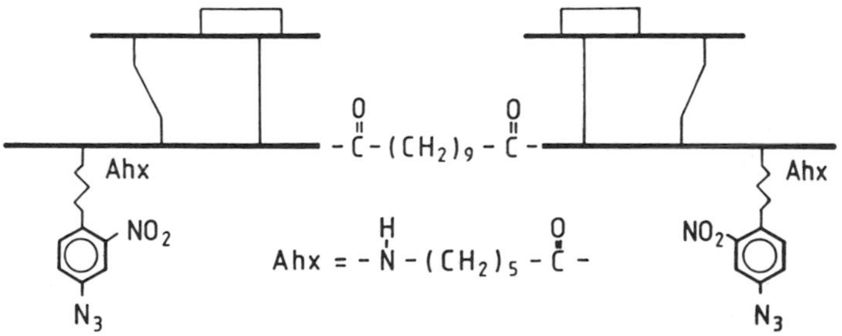

FIG.5. Structure of the dimeric, bivalent photo-insulin (1,2).

It was prepared by linking two   A1,B29-Msc-insulins
through their B1-amino groups with azelaic acid bis-p-
nitrophenylester according to ref. 47.   Removal of Msc
groups was followed by selective re-acylation with Msc
groups at the A1-amino groups.   Then, the photoreactive
groups were introduced into both B29 positions (yield:
85%).   After deblocking, preparative HPLC yielded the
bivalent photo-insulin. It contains crosslink and photo
groups in an arrangement which is not cleavable by
thiols. Thus, the covalent complexes formed after
photo-affinity labelling of receptors can be analyzed
by SDS/PAGE also under reducing conditions.
    Preliminary experiments showed that the affinity for
receptors under reversible conditions is somewhat lower
than expected, but it should be sufficient for covalent
binding studies.
    In this work, extensive use was made of HPLC on
reversed phase, and dimeric insulins were characterized
by this technique for the first time. An example is
shown in Figure 6.   Msc-insulin dimers are well differentiated with respect to site and number of Msc-groups.
Desamido components, which are present in most insulin
preparations, are only partially resolved (shoulders on
the right side). The retention time of monomeric
insulin is about 10 minutes, of the photo-dimer about
40 minutes under similar conditions.

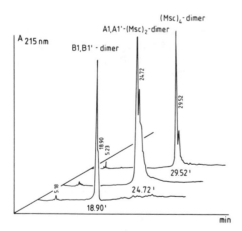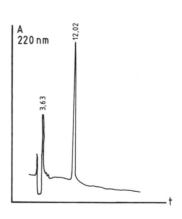

FIG.6. Left: HPLC of dimeric insulins on Nucleosil
7 C18 in ammonium dihydrogen phosphate/acetonitrile, pH
3.0 (linear gradient) (1).
Right: HPLC of B29-(Nap-Lys(Biot))insulin on Lichrosorb
5 C18 in triethylammonium phosphate/acetonitrile (linear gradient) (54).

Photo-reactive proinsulin
In order to test our assumption that locking
molecules with low affinity at the receptor site might
enhance efficacy, bovine proinsulin (a gift of B.
Frank) was acylated with the Abz-group. Preferential
substitution at the terminal amino group occurred at
low pH, and homogeneous 1-Abz-proinsulin was isolated
by preparative HPLC (53).

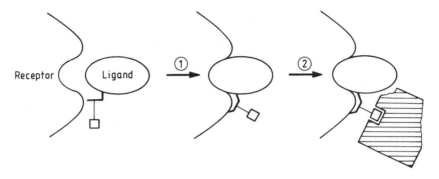

FIG. 7. Principle of photo-affinity mediated complexing
(PAMAC) (54)

A new principle for receptor analysis
To broaden the scope of photo-affinity labelling
even more, we combined it with another powerful technique, biotin-avidin complexing (review: 6), which has
very successfully been applied to insulin and its receptor (18). As outlined in Figure 7, the ligand, which
carries a hetero-bifunctional reactive site, is first
cross-linked to the receptor by irradiation. In the
second step a reversible complex with soluble or car-
rier-bound avidin (also derivatized avidin and strept-
avidin, 18) can be formed and subsequently isolated.
The lysine derivative (Fig.4) was attached to the
B29 group of A1,B1-protected insulin. After deblocking,
HPLC yielded the desired insulin (Table, Fig.6). Iodination and subsequent HPLC gave the B26-monoiodo derivative. UV-induced linking to receptors of human
placenta and adipocytes showed, after SDS/PAGE and
autoradiography, the familiar pattern of bands, corresponding to the tetramer and the α-subunit.
The crucial question was whether avidin would bind
to the complex. When the band containing the α-subunit
was transferred from one electrophoretogram to another
gel and re-run in the presence of succinyl-avidin, its
position was shifted from M_r 130.000 to a new position,
corresponding to M_r 161.000. In the presence of excess
biotin, the mobility was unchanged. This finding
clearly demonstrated formation of the ternary complex

and the applicability of our concept.
The new 125-I-labelled insulin derivative contains all the essentials for fingerprint analysis of the insulin-binding site of the receptor:
    a) satisfactory receptor affinity and biopotency,
    b) a single cleavage site for trypsin (B22-Arg),
    c) radioactivity in the insulin fragment remaining linked to receptor fragments (B26-Tyr), and
    d) the biotin residue for "fishing" the desired fragments at all stages of the analytical process. The analysis of human placental receptor is currently under investigation (F. Wedekind, 54).

CONCLUSIONS

Insulins with altered structure and specific modifications are important for fundamental and application-oriented diabetes research. The rapid development of recombinant DNA-technology has provided human insulin for treatment, and also a first series of analogues (35). However, many of the insulins described in this paper cannot be obtained via genetic techniques. Thus, the approaches are complementary. A sensible combination of methods will - in the future - lead to further variants necessary to answer the many open questions, and possibly provide insulins with improved therapeutic properties.

ACKNOWLEDGEMENT

We thank for financial support: DFG (SFB 113), EC (Stimulation Action) and Ministerium für Wissenschaft und Forschung NRW. We are grateful to all friends and colleagues who participated in the collaborative projects mentioned , and to H. Zahn and H. Höcker for their constant interest and encouragement.

REFERENCES

1. Ambrosius, D. (1985): Diploma Thesis, TH Aachen.
2. Ambrosius, D., Bala-Mohan, S., Behrendt, C., Schäfer, K., Schüttler, A., and Brandenburg, D. (1987): In: Peptides, edited by Theodoropoulos, pp. 521-523. Walter de Gruyter, Berlin, New York.
3. Behrendt, C. (1986): Diploma Thesis, TH Aachen
4. Berhanu, P., Saunders, D.J., and Brandenburg, D. (1987): Biochem. J., 242: 589-596.
5. Bi, R.C., Dauter, Z., Dodson, E., Dodson, G., Gordiano, F., and Reynolds, C. (1984): Biopolymers, 23: 391-395.
6. Billingsley, M.L., Pennypacker, K.R., Hoover, C.G., and Kincaid, R.L. (1987): Biotechniques, 5: 22-31.

7. Blundell, T., and Wood, S. (1982): Ann. Rev. Biochem., 51: 123-154.
8. Brandenburg, D. (1981): In: Medicinal Chemistry Advances, edited by F.G. de las Heras and S. Vega, pp. 487-502. Pergamon Press, Oxford, New York.
9. Brandenburg, D., Saunders, D., and Schüttler, A. (1983): In: Amino-acids, Peptides and Proteins: Specialist Periodical Reports, Senior Reporter J.H. Jones, Vol. 14, pp. 461-476. Royal Society of Chemistry, London.
10. Brandenburg, D., Diaconescu, C., Klotz, G., Mucke, P., Neffe, J., Saunders, D., and Schüttler, A. (1985): Biochimie, 67: 1111-1117.
11. Casaretto, M., Spoden, M., Diaconescu, C., Gattner, H.-G., Zahn, H., Brandenburg, D., and Wollmer, A. (1987): Biol. Chem. Hoppe-Seyler, 368: 709-717.
12. Chap, Z., Ishida, T., Chou, J. Hartley, C.J., Entman, M.L., Brandenburg, D., Jones, R.H., and Field, J.B. (1987): Am. J. Physiol., 252: E209-E217.
13. Ciaraldi, T., Robbins, R., Leidy, J.W., Thamm, P., and Berhanu, P. (1985): Endocrinology, 116: 2179-2185.
14. Deger, A., Krämer, H., Rapp, R., Koch, R., and Weber, U. (1986): Biochem. Biophys. Res. Comm., 135: 458-464.
15. Diaconescu, C., Saunders, D., Gattner, H.-G., and Brandenburg, D. (1982): Hoppe-Seylers Z. Physiol. Chem., 363: 187-192.
16. Fehlmann, M., Chvatchko, Y., Brandenburg, D., Van Obberghen, E., and Brossette, N. (1985): Biochimie, 67: 1155-1159.
17. Fehlmann, M., Peyron, J.-F., Samson, M., Van Obberghen, E., Brandenburg, D., and Brossette, N. (1985): Proc. Natl. Acad. Sci. USA, 82: 8634-8637.
18. Finn, F.M., Titus, G., Horstman, D., and Hofmann, K. (1984): Proc. Natl. Acad. Sci. USA, 81: 7328-7332.
19. Fischer, W.H., Saunders, D., Brandenburg, D., Diaconescu, C., Wollmer, A., Dodson, G., De Meyts, P., and Zahn, H. (1986): Biol. Chem. Hoppe-Seyler, 367: 999-1006.
20. Fischer, W.H., Saunders, D., Brandenburg, D., Wollmer, A., and Zahn, H. (1985): Biol. Chem. Hoppe-Seyler, 366: 521-525.
21. Fischer, W.H., Saunders, D.J., Zahn, H., and Wollmer, A. (1985): In: Peptides: Structure and Function, edited by C.M. Deber, V.J. Hruby, and K.D. Kopple, pp. 301-304.Pierce Chemical Company, Rockford, Illinois.
22. Gammeltoft, S. (1984): Physiol. Rev.,64: 1321-78.

23. Gattner, H.-G., Danho, W., Knorr, R., and Zahn, H. (1982): In: Chemistry of Peptides and Proteins, Vol. 1, edited by W. Voelter, E. Wünsch, Y. Ovchinnikov, and V. Ivanov, pp. 319-325. Walter de Gruyter, Berlin, New York.
24. Gattner, H.-G., and Leithäuser, M. (1986): In: Chemistry of Peptides and Proteins, Vol. 3, edited by W. Voelter, E. Bayer, Y.A. Ovchinnikov, and V.T Ivanov, pp. 99-104. W.de Gruyter, Berlin, New York
25. Gazzano, H., Halban, P., Prentki, M., Ballotti, R., Brandenburg, D., Fehlmann, M., and Van Obberghen, E. (1985): Biochem. J., 226: 867-872.
26. Heidenreich, K.A., and Brandenburg, D. (1986): Endocrinology, 118: 1835-1842.
27. Hueckstaedt, T., J.M. Olefsky, D. Brandenburg, and K.A. . Heidenreich (1986): J. Biol. Chem., 261: 8655-8659.
28. Juul, S.M., Jones, R.H., Evans, J.L., Neffe, J., Sönksen P., and Brandenburg, D. (1986): Biochim. Biophys. Acta, 856: 310-319.
29. Juul, S.M., Neffe, J., Evans, J.L., Jones, R.H., Sönksen, P.H., and Brandenburg, D. (1986): Biochim. Biophys. Acta, 856: 320-324.
30. Kahn, C.R. (1985): Ann. Rev. Med.,36: 429-451.
31. King, G.L., Kahn, C.R., Samuels, B., Danho, W., Bullesbach, E.E., and Gattner, H.G. (1982): J. Biol. Chem., 257: 10869-10873.
32. Knorr, R., Danho, W., Büllesbach, E.E., Gattner, H.-G., and Zahn, H. (1983): Hoppe-Seylers Z. Physiol. Chem., 364: 1615-1626.
33. Knorr, R., Danho, W., Büllesbach, E.E., Gattner, H.-G., Zahn, H., King, G.L., and Kahn, C.R. (1982): Hoppe- Seylers Z. Physiol. Chem., 363: 1449-1460.
34. Kobayashi, M., Ohgaku, S., Iwasaki, M., Maegawa, H., Shigeta, Y., and Inouye, K. (1982): Biochem. Biophys. Res. Comm., 107: 329-336.
35. Markussen, J., Diers, I., Engesgaard, A., Hansen, M.T. Hougaard, P., Langkjaer, L., Norris, K., Ribel, U., Sorensen, A.R., Sorensen, E., and Voigt, H.O.(1987): Protein Engineering, 1: 215-223
36. Mucke, P., Diaconescu, C., Klotz, G., Jorgensen, P., Saunders, D., and Brandenburg, D. (1987): Biol. Chem. Hoppe-Seyler, 368: 85-92.
37. Naithani, V.K., and Gattner, H.G. (1982): Hoppe-Seylers Z. Physiol. Chem., 363: 1443-1448.
38. Nakagawa, S.H., and Tager, H.S. (1986): J. Biol. Chem., 261: 7332-7341.
39. Offord, R.E. (1987): Prot. Engineering, 1: 151-157
40. Peyron, J.F., Samson, M., Van Obberghen, E., Brandenburg, D., and Fehlmann, M. (1985): Diabetologia, 28: 369-372.

41. Podlecki, D.A., Smith, R.M., Kao, M., Tsai, P., Hueckstaedt, T., Brandenburg, D., Lasher, R.S., Jarett, L., and Olefsky, J.M. (1987): J. Biol. Chem., 262: 3362-3368.
42. Roth, R.A., Cassell, D.J., Morgan, D.O., Tatnell, M.A., Jones, R.H., Schüttler, A., and Brandenburg, D. (1984): FEBS Lett., 170: 360-364.
43. Saunders, D., and Brandenburg, D. (1984): In: Methods in Diabetes Research, Vol. I: Laboratory Methods, Part A, edited by J. Larner and S. Pohl, pp. 3-22. John Wiley, New York.
44. Saunders, D., and Freude, K (1982): Hoppe-Seylers Z. Physiol. Chem., 363: 655-659.
45. Saunders, D., Freude, K., Naithani, V.K., and Brandenburg, D. (1983): In: Peptides 1982, edited by K. Blaha and P. Malon, pp. 371-374. Walter de Gruyter, Berlin, New York.
46. Schartmann, B., Gattner, H.-G., Danho, W., and Zahn, H. (1983): Hoppe-Seylers Z. Physiol. Chem., 364: 179-186.
47. Schüttler, A., and Brandenburg, D. (1982): Hoppe-Seylers Z. Physiol. Chem., 363: 317-330.
48. Schüttler, A., Diaconescu, C., Saunders, D.J., and Brandenburg, D. (1985): Biochem. J., 232: 49-53.
49. Schüttler, A., Gattner, H.-G., and Brandenburg, D. (1984): In: Methods in Diabetes Research, Vol. I: Laboratory Methods, Part B, edited by J. Larner and S. Pohl, pp. 355-376. John Wiley, New York.
50. Tanti, J.-F., Gremeaux, T., Brandenburg, D., Van Obberghen, E., and Le Marchand-Brustel, Y. (1986): Diabetes, 35: 1243-1248.
51. Tatnell, M.A., Jones, R.H, Willey,K.P. Schüttler, A. and D. Brandenburg (1983): Biochem. J., 216: 687-694.
52. Trindler, P., and Brandenburg, D. (1982): In: Chemistry of Peptides and Proteins, Vol. 1, edited by W. Voelter, E. Wünsch, Yu. Ovchinnikov, and V. Ivanov, pp.308-314. W.de Gruyter, Berlin, New York
53. Van de Löcht-Blasberg, M. (1987): Diploma Thesis, TH Aachen.
54. Wedekind, F., Thesis RWTH Aachen, in preparation.
55. Wieneke, H.-J., Danho, W., Büllesbach, E.E., Gattner, H.-G., and Zahn, H. (1983): Hoppe-Seylers Z. Physiol. Chem., 364: 537-550.
56. Wieneke, H.-J., Wolf, G., Wolff, W., Büllesbach, E.E., Gattner, H.-G., and Brandenburg, D. (1983): In: Peptides 1982, edited by K. Blaha and P. Malon, pp. 367-370. W.de Gruyter, Berlin, New York
57. Yip, C.C., and Yeung, C.W.T. (1985): Methods Enzymol., 109: 170-179.

Insulin Action and Diabetes,
edited by H. Joseph Goren et al.
Raven Press, New York © 1988.

THE COVALENT TAGGING OF THE CELL SURFACE INSULIN RECEPTOR
WITH THE GENERATION OF AN INSULIN-FREE RECEPTOR

Victoria P. Knutson

The University of Texas Health Science Center at Houston
Medical School, Department of Pharmacology
Houston, Texas 77225

Good morning everybody. One of the primary interests in my
laboratory is the catabolic processing of the insulin receptor.
In particular, we are investigating the basal and hormonally-
modified recycling of the insulin receptor and its inactivation
and degradation. To pursue these studies we wanted to have a
method to specifically tag the insulin receptor in such a way
that the ligand was not covalently attached to the insulin-
receptor complex. The rationale to this madness was that in
the normal processing of the insulin receptor, insulin is
discharged from the complex at some time during the lifetime of
the insulin receptor. Therefore, any crosslinking agent that
would covalently attach insulin to its receptor may significantly perturb the normal processing of the insulin receptor
itself. About the time that we were trying to figure out some
method to achieve this tagging of the insulin receptor, a
hetero-bifunctional crosslinking reagent became commercially
available. This hetero-bifunctional reagent had an N-hydroxysuccinimide ester on one end of it, which could be easily
displaced for coupling to ligand. On the other end of the
reagent was an arylazide moiety, which, by photolysis, enables
the attachment of crosslinking reagent to the receptor. This
reagent, which has the acronym SASD, differs from hetero-
bifunctional reagents which had been used up to this point in
that the two ends of this reagent were separated by a disulfide
bond. Upon reduction of this disulfide bond, the ligand end of
the reagent would separate from the end of the reagent that was
crosslinked to the receptor. In addition, the arylazide part
of the reagent, the part that would be attached to the receptor, could be iodinated. Therefore, we could potentially introduce a small molecular weight moiety photolytically into the
insulin receptor with a radioactive tag, which could ultimately
be discharged from insulin itself.

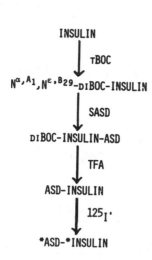

FIG. 1. The coupling of insulin to SASD. Details of the sequence are described in the text. tBOC, t-butoxycarbonyl; TFA, trifluoroacetic acid. Reproduced from Knutson (2) with permission from The Journal of Biological Chemistry.

Figure 1 is a schematic of the method by which we have been coupling insulin to the SASD molecule with subsequent iodination. As shown in this figure, insulin is modified with the blocking agent t-butoxycarbonyl on the alpha amino group of A1 glycine and the epsilon amino group of B29 lysine to generate diBOC-insulin, as described by Geiger et al. (1). SASD, the hetero-bifunctional agent, is then added to the purified diBOC-insulin with resultant displacement of N-hydroxysuccinimide group from the SASD. The product is diBOC-insulin with the azido portion of the probe attached to insulin. Trifluoroacetic acid will remove the two BOC residues, resulting in the formation of the photoprobe ASD-insulin. Iodination at this point results in the incorporation of ^{125}I-iodine into both the insulin moiety and the arylazide moiety. This probe, ^{125}I-ASD-insulin, will bind to the cell surface insulin receptor with the same characteristic binding affinity and capacity as radiolabeled insulin itself. In addition, we have found that we get approximately equimolar incorporation of ^{125}I into both the ASD part of the molecule and into the insulin part of the molecule.

Figure 2 is a schematic of the coupling of the ASD-insulin molecule to the insulin receptor. When ASD-insulin is added to the receptor, we get the noncovalent association of ASD-insulin with the receptor. Upon photolysis with ultraviolet light, a covalent bond attaches the ASD part of the molecule to the receptor. At this point, mild reduction with the reducing agent glutathione results in the release of the insulin-containing portion of the molecule from the receptor and the maintenance of the iodinated small probe attached to the receptor molecule. The photolysis step is time- and pH-dependent and we can achieve on the average 15-20% occupancy of the cell-surface receptor with the probe. The glutathione reduction is concentration- and time-dependent. We can achieve essentially total release of the insulin moiety from the cell surface receptor. The general metabolic state of the cell is not

compromised by this multiple treatment, as assessed by the
incorporation of leucine into cellular protein, insulin degradation and glucose and amino acid uptake in both the basal and
insulin-stimulated states.

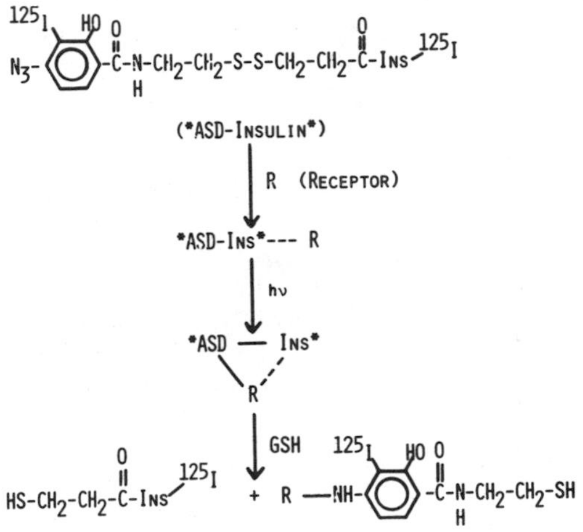

FIG. 2. The coupling of ASD-insulin to the cell surface
insulin receptor. Details of the sequence are described in
the text. R, receptor; GSH, reduced glutathione; - - -,
noncovalent bond; ——, covalent bond. Reproduced from Knutson (2) with permission from The Journal of Biological
Chemistry.

In conclusion, we have found that it is possible to label
the cell surface insulin receptor in a manner that is specific,
which does not seem to perturb the general cellular metabolism,
and most importantly, allows for the release of insulin from
the labelled receptor.

This work was been supported by grant number AM35397 from
The National Institutes of Health. A full description of this
work has been published (2).

REFERENCES

1. Geiger, R., Schone, H.-H., and Pfaff, W. (1971): J. Phys.
   Chem., 352:1487-1490.

2. Knutson, V.P. (1987): J. Biol. Chem., 262:2374-2383.

Insulin Action and Diabetes,
edited by H. Joseph Goren et al.
Raven Press, New York © 1988.

CELL SURFACE INSULIN RECEPTOR COMPLEX

C.C. Yip, M.L. Moule, and M.L. Phillips

Banting and Best Department of Medical Research,
University of Toronto, Toronto, Ontario
Canada M5G 1L6

As the title of my presentation suggests, I am going to talk about the complexity of the insulin receptor on the cell surface. As Dr. Rutter mentioned in his presentation, the insulin receptor is composed of the alpha and beta subunit and possibly exists as a tetramer on the cell membrane. However, the insulin receptor may be a little more complicated than that. From our studies it seems that the insulin receptor on the cell membrane is in association with some other membrane components. In this particular case, I want to tell you about the association of the insulin receptor with Class I transplantation antigens and hopefully to give you some idea of what we are thinking about the functional significance of this association. My colleagues, Dr. Laurie Phillips and Dr. Margaret Moule are the main contributors to the work I am presenting here.

Dr. Brandenburg's presentation provided a background description of the process of making photoreactive insulin to label the insulin receptor. My laboratory was one of the first to apply this technique when we started to study the insulin receptor. In our work we have consistently observed photo-labelling of receptor components that we believe to be smaller than the designated alpha and beta subunits; particularly a component of about 45 kDa (6). This is not a degradation product, rather we have obtained data strongly suggesting that the 45-kDa receptor components are likely the Class I transplantation antigens (4). These antigens are composed of the K, D, and L gene products (M_r about 45 kDa) of the major histocompatibility complex ($H-2$) of mouse chromosome 17. On the cell surface, each of them is in association with a peptide of 12 kDa, called β_2-microglobulin, which is coded by a different gene on a different chromosome (5). The extracellular domains of these antigens are highly polymorphic, and different strains of inbred animals have different haplotypes. In our studies we examined the association of Class I antigens with the insulin receptor in mice of the k, b and s haplotypes (Table I).

TABLE 1.   Mouse Strains and Their Haplotypes

Strain	Haplotype	K	A	E	D
C3H	k	k	k	k	k
BALB.B	b	b	b	b	b
Bl0.S	s	s	s	s	s

The A and E are Class II antigens which are not associated with the insulin receptor. As shown in the Table, the C3H strain of mice has a k haplotype for both for both the K and the D antigens. Antibodies to the Class I transplantation antigens are haplotype specific. Thus, for example, antibodies against H-2K^K, i.e. against the K antigen of C3H mice, do not react with the H-2K^B, i.e. the K antigen of BALB.B mice.

In our studies, we use the technique of photoaffinity labelling and immunoprecipitation by specific antibodies to demonstrate the association between these antigens and the insulin receptor. We used two separate approaches in our experiments as outlined below:

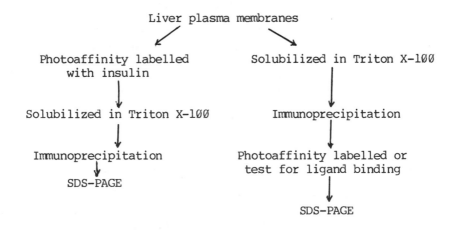

Figure 1 shows the results of an experiment using the prephotolabelling technique and immunoprecipitation with a

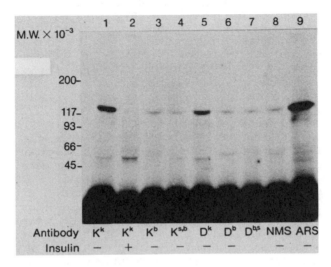

Fig. 1. Liver plasma membranes were prepared from C3H mice. Photoaffinity labelling and immunoprecipitation were carried out as described (4). NMS: normal mouse serum, ARS: anti-receptor serum, Ab indicates antibody used: e.g. K^k, antibody to the K antigen of k haplotype, In(+): an excess of insulin was present during binding and photolysis to establish specificity of photolabelling. The photolabelled receptor subunit is indicated by solid square.

monoclonal antibody against H-2K^k. Membranes used were prepared from C3H (H-2^k) mice. Precipitation by anti-receptor antibody (ARS) brought down insulin receptor as evidenced by the presence of the labelled β subunit of the receptor (lane 9). Normal mouse serum precipitation showed no band (lane 8). The antibody against K^k also clearly brought down the insulin receptor as shown by the presence of the photolabelled subunit (lane 1). In contrast, an antibody against K^b, that is, a different haplotype but the same antigen K, did not precipitate the insulin receptor (lane 3). Antibody against D^k, that is the D antigen of k haplotype also immunoprecipitated the insulin receptor in the liver plasma membranes of C3H mice (lane 5). Similar haplotype specific immunoprecipitation of insulin receptors was obtained when we used liver plasma membranes prepared from BALB.B mice of b haplotype and from B10.S mice of s haplotype. The insulin receptor is also precipitated by antibody to the β_2-microglobulin (data not shown).

Now the question is: are all the insulin receptors on the liver plasma membrane associated with the Class I antigen? Figure 1 shows that the precipitation by the anti-receptor antibody brought down much more photolabelled insulin receptor than either one of the monoclonal antibodies against the Class I antigens. We carried out double immunoprecipitation experiments to answer this question. Results obtained are shown in Figure 2. In lane 1 (Figure 2) you can see the precipitation of the insulin receptor by ARS, and in lane 2 by anti-K^k; and in lane 4 the supernatant from the precipitation with ARS was re-precipitated with the anti-K^k resulting in the precipitation of a trace of the labelled receptor. In contrast, when the supernatant from the precipitation with anti-K^k was treated with ARS, more insulin receptors were precipitated (lane 6). Up to this point the data suggest that not all the insulin receptors on the plasma membrane of the liver are in association with Class I antigens. Only a small proportion of them is in association with Class I antigens. More importantly the last panel of this figure shows that when we precipitated with anti-K^k, i.e. to bring down the insulin receptor with an antibody against one of the two antigens, in this case the K antigen, and then re-precipitated with the antibody against D^k, i.e. the other antigen, we could no longer bring down any more photolabelled receptors (lane 9). When we precipitated with anti-D^k and then re-precipitated with anti-K^k, no more receptor was precipitated. The results show

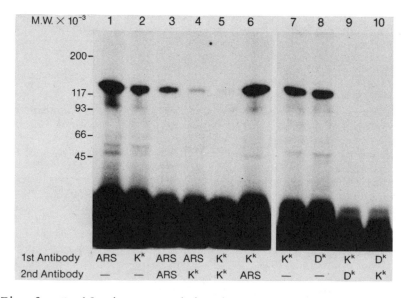

Fig. 2. Double immunoprecipitation of solubilized photo-labelled insulin receptors. Supernatant obtained after precipitation with the first antibody was re-precipitated with the second antibody as indicated.

that antibodies against any one of the two antigens, K or D, precipitated all the receptors that were in association with the Class I antigens. Thus it appears that those insulin receptors that are precipitated with antibodies against Class I transplantation antigens are associated with both the K and the D antigens in the same complex. Since antibodies to β_2-microglobulin also precipitated the insulin receptor, the receptor appears to be in association with the entire Class I H-2 complex.

The next question is: is the insulin receptor unique in its association with the Class I antigens?. To answer this question we carried out experiments using the other approach outlined above: precipitating the receptor first and then examining the binding of the ligand to the immunoprecipitate.

We precipitated solubilized liver plasma membrane with antibody against K^K or with anti-receptor antibody and then determined if the immune complex could bind the ligand. There was hardly any insulin binding by the precipitate obtained with normal mouse serum (Figure 3). The immunoprecipitate obtained with anti-K^K exhibited a high degree of insulin binding, demonstrating that the association that we observed was not induced by the binding of insulin to the receptor. In the photolabelling experiment one can argue that the association may have been the result of insulin binding to the receptor, inducing the association. Here, there was no insulin binding to begin with and insulin binding was demonstrated after we precipitated the complex. Figure 3 also shows that insulin binding to the anti-receptor precipitates was lower than that obtained with the anti-K^K precipitates. This was expected because this anti-receptor antibody inhibits insulin binding. The other ligand we looked at was epidermal growth factor (EGF). Interestingly, EGF also bound specifically to the precipitates obtained with anti-K^K. In contrast, the immunoprecipitate obtained with anti-receptor antibody was not able to bind EGF at all. When we precipitated the soluble membrane with anti-receptor antibody first and then re-precipitated the supernatant with anti-K^K, the binding of EGF to the precipitates was unchanged while insulin binding was greatly reduced as expected. These observations indicate that, in addition to insulin receptor, possibly the EGF receptor is also in association with Class I transplantation antigens on the cell membrane. Using this approach, we found that neither the glucagon receptor nor the receptor for atrial natriuretic factor was associated with Class I transplantation antigens.

Now the question is: what is the significance of such an association? Does it mean anything? We began by asking whether the association might be involved in the regulation of

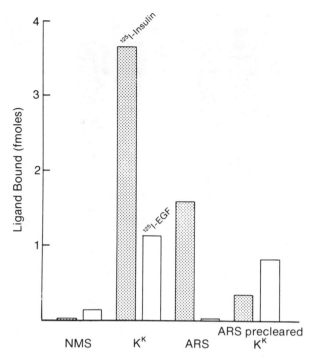

Fig. 3. Solubilized liver plasma membranes from C3H mice were immunoprecipitated with normal mouse serum (NMS) antibody to H-2K^K or anti-receptor serum (ARS). Binding of ^{125}I-labelled insulin or EGF to the immune complex was measured as described (4).

the receptor tyrosine kinase activity. What we did was to solubilize the membrane and then carry out the experiment by two methods. In the first method, we immunoprecipitated the receptor first, and then allowed the immunoprecipitate to undergo phosphorylation in the presence or absence of insulin. We then analyzed the immunoprecipitate for insulin receptor autophosphorylation. In the second method the autophosphorylation of the insulin receptor was allowed to occur and then the phosphorylated receptors were precipitated with either the anti-receptor antibody or the anti-Class I antibody. Figure 4 shows the result obtained with the first method. Phosphorylation of the 95-kDa   subunit of the receptor occurred in the precipitates obtained with the anti-receptor antibody. The reason why the receptor phosphorylation in this case did not appear to be stimulated by insulin was that this anti-receptor antibody can mimic the action of insulin. As a control, there was no receptor phosphorylation in the precipitate obtained with normal serum. But interestingly enough, no receptor phosphorylation occurred in the preci-

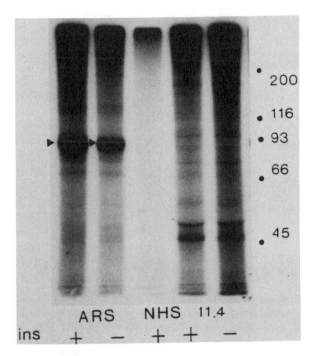

Fig. 4. Solubilized liver plasma membranes from C3H mice were immunoprecipitated with anti-receptor$_k$ antibody (ARS), normal human immunoglobulin (NHS) and anti-k^k antibody (11.4). The immunoprecipitates were incubated with insulin (+) and then with ^{32}P-ATP and Mn^{++}. The phosphorylated β subunit is indicated (▶).

pitate obtained with the anti-K^k monoclonal antibody either.

Figure 5 shows the results obtained using the second method, i.e. phosphorylating the soluble receptor first and then immunoprecipitating with anti-receptor antibody or the anti-Class I antibody. The results show that, as expected, insulin stimulated the phosphorylation of the subunit which was precipitated by the anti-receptor antibody. In contrast, like normal serum used as a control, the monoclonal antibody against Class I again did not precipitate the insulin receptors that were phosphorylated. It was important for us to determine that it was not something in the anti-Class I monoclonal antibody that might have dephosphorylated the receptor. The last lane in this figure shows that when we mixed the anti-Class I antibody with the anti-receptor antibody together, there was precipitation of the phosphorylated receptor as evidenced by

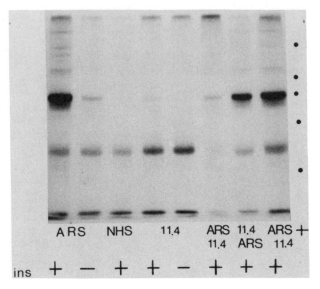

Fig. 5. Solubilized liver plasma membranes from C3H mice were incubated with insulin and phosphorylated with ^{32}P-ATP and Mn^{++}. The reaction was stopped and antibody was added as indicated. For lanes 6 and 7, the supernatant from the first precipitation was re-precipitated with the antibody indicated. For lane 8, anti-receptor antibody and anti-K^k antibody were added together.

the detection of the phosphorylated β subunit. The results of these experiments show that the anti-receptor antibody clearly can, as expected, immunoprecipitate phosphorylated receptors, but the anti-K^k monoclonal antibody apparently cannot. In spite of the fact that the anti-K^k antibody can precipitate photolabelled insulin receptors and in spite of the fact that it can precipitate receptors that can bind insulin, it is not able to recognize or to immunoprecipitate receptors that can undergo autophosphorylation.

In conclusion, I would like to suggest that a proportion of the insulin receptors on the cell membrane exists as a complex in association with the K and D Class I antigens. This association has also been observed by other investigators recently (1-3). From the data that we have obtained on phosphorylation, it would seem that insulin receptors in association with the Class I antigens are lacking in their ability to undergo autophosphorylation.

References
1. Due, C., Simonsen, M., and Olsson, L.C. (1986): Proc. Natl. Acad. Sci. USA 83: 6007-6011.
2. Fehlmann, M., Peyron, J.R., Samson, M., van Obberghen, E., Brandenburg, D., and Brossette, N. (1985): Proc. Natl. Acad. Sci. USA, 82: 8634-8637.
3. Kittur, D., Shimizu, Y., DeMars, R., and Edidin, M. (1987): Proc. Natl. Acad. Sci. USA, 84: 1351-1355.
4. Phillips, M.L., Moule, M.L., Delovitch, T.L., and Yip, C.C. (1986): Proc. Natl. Acad. Sci. USA, 83: 3747-3478.
5. Steinmetz, M., and Hood, L. (1983): Science, 222: 727-733.
6. Yip, C.C., and Moule, M.L. (1983): Diabetes, 32: 760-767.

Acknowledgement
This study was supported by a grant from the Canadian Diabetes Association, and from the Medical Research Council.

Insulin Action and Diabetes,
edited by H. Joseph Goren et al.
Raven Press, New York © 1988.

REGULATION OF THE INSULIN RECEPTOR
BY MULTI-SITE PHOSPHORYLATION

C. Ronald Kahn, S. Sethu K. Reddy,
Steve Shoelson, H. Joseph Goren[*], and Morris F. White

Research Division, Joslin Diabetes Center,
Department of Medicine, Harvard Medical School,
Boston, Massachusetts USA 02215
[*]Department of Biochemistry, University of Calgary,
Calgary, Alberta Canada T2N 4N1

The insulin receptor is a transmembranous heterotetrameric glycoprotein composed of two α- and two β-subunits (8). The α-subunit with a molecular weight of 135,000 Daltons, contains the insulin binding domain and the β-subunit with a molecular weight of 95,000 Daltons contains a protein tyrosine kinase (7). Insulin binding to the α-subunit activates the tyrosine kinase resulting in insulin receptor autophosphorylation which may initiate a chain of events leading to insulin action (6).

The insulin receptor kinase has been shown to be homologous to many other tyrosine kinases (3,11). Like these other kinases, many of which are retroviral oncogene products, ATP is the unique phosphate donor and Mn^{2+} is a necessary cofactor. The receptor kinase can phosphorylate the β-subunit as well as exogenous substrates (1,9,12,14). Phosphorylation occurs exclusively on tyrosine residues in a cell-free system but in intact cells, autophosphorylation may be seen on serines as well. Insulin increases the V_{max} of the kinase and divalent cations such as Mn^{2+} and Mg^{2+} alter the K_m. The autophosphorylation state of the insulin receptor has been shown to be another important regulator of kinase activity by several groups (6,9,12,14). This autoactivation of the kinase and amplification process occur over several minutes and is slow when compared to the rapid actions of insulin.

We have tried to determine the sites of autophosphorylation in the β-subunit and to also distinguish which of these sites

43

result in autoactivation of the receptor kinase. The amino acids in the β-subunit will be numbered according to the sequence deduced by Ullrich et al; the sequence determined by Rutter's group contains an extra 12 amino acids but the β-subunits are otherwise identical. Important domains therefore include the lysine residue at 1118 position (ATP binding site) and two tyrosines at 953 and 960, three tyrosines clustered near 1150, and a group of two tyrosines at 1316 and 1322 (possible auto-phosphorylation sites).

C-terminal Domain: Our first approach was to use limited proteolytic digestion combined with peptide mapping and immunoprecipitation with various antibodies to specific domains of the β-subunit. When the β-subunit is labelled with ^{32}P-ATP and is then subjected to very low concentrations of trypsin for up to 10 minutes, the β-subunit undergoes sequential proteolytic cleavage to an 85 Kd and then to 70 Kd fragments. Within one minute, virtually all of the 95 Kd subunit is cleaved to the 85 Kd fragment which contains only 70% of the total radioactivity incorporated into the 95 Kd β-subunit during autophosphorylation (Fig. 1).

Tryptic peptide mapping of the various fragments using reverse phase HPLC was performed (Fig. 2). The 95 Kd subunit has three major sites denoted as pY1, pY2 and pY3 and two minor sites denoted as pY1a and pY4. Mapping of the 85 Kd fragment revealed that pY2 and pY3 are almost completely lost. Thus the missing 10Kd fragment contains two possible phosphorylation sites.

Examination of the β-subunit sequence suggested that there was a trypsin sensitive site in the C-terminal which could result in the 85Kd and 10 Kd fragments. A peptide antibody raised against the C-terminal domain containing the 1316 and 1322 tyrosines was used to immunoprecipitate the 95 Kd intact β-subunit and the 85 Kd fragment. The antibody failed to recognize the 85 Kd fragment confirming the hypothesis of the 10 Kd fragment to be originating from the C-terminal.

Another way to confirm this hypothesis was to separate radioactively labelled peaks pY2 and pY3 and to perform amino acid sequenation in a liquid phase sequenator (in collaboration with H. Keutman, Mass. General Hospital). By analyzing the number of radioactive peaks (two peaks) and the distance between the peaks (six amino acids), we deduced that the data was consistent with the 10 Kd fragment containing the 1316 and 1322 tyrosines.

Are these the sites responsible for activation of the tyrosine kinase activity? The 95 Kd intact β-subunit and the 85 Kd fragment both have full kinase activity when comparing their ability to phosphorylate a synthetic exogenous peptide (Fig. 3).

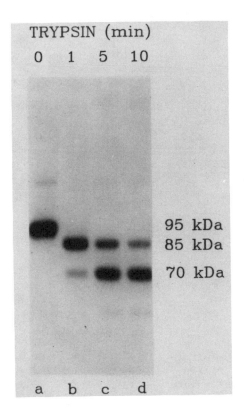

FIGURE 1: Time course of trypsin treatment of prephos-
phorylated insulin receptor. Partially purified insulin
receptor was phosphorylated with ^{32}P-ATP and then digested
with low concentration of trypsin. The reaction was
terminated and the receptor was then reduced with DTT and
separated by SDS-PAGE. There is rapid cleavage of the intact
95 kDa subunit to an 85 kDa fragment and subsequently a 70 kDa
fragment. Lane a (0 min), lane b (1 min), lane c (5 min) and
lane d (10 min).

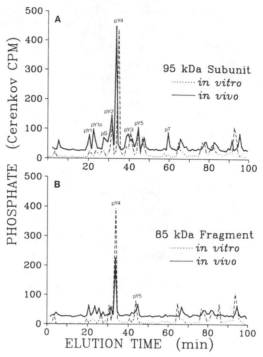

FIGURE 2: Analysis of the in vitro and in vivo autophosphorylation sites in the β-subunit of the insulin receptor
by tryptic peptide mapping. The receptor was separated by
SDS-PAGE and then digested completely with trypsin. The
resulting phosphopeptides were separated by reverse phase
HPLC. The phosphotyrosine peaks are denoted pY1, pY1a, pY2,
pY3, pY4 and pY5. Phosphoserine (pS) and phosphothreonine
(pT) peaks are also noted. Differences between in vitro and
in vivo autophosphorylation as well as differences between the
95 kDa subunit and the 85 kDa fragment are shown. See Text
for details.

So it appears that although the C-terminal is autophosphorylated, it is not required for the autoactivation
phenomenon.

First Autophosphorylation Site: We thought that perhaps the
first site of autophosphorylation may be important in activation
of the kinase. To study this aspect of receptor autophosphorylation , antiphosphotyrosine antibodies, raised in rabbits
injected with Keyhole Limpet Hemocyanin coupled to phospho-
tyramine, were used to immunoprecipitate the phosphorylated
insulin receptor. More importantly, these antibodies should
trap the first phosphorylated form of the insulin receptor and
prevent further autophosphorylation. In fact, we observed that
in the presence of the phosphotyrosine antibodies, autophosphorylation of the receptor was inhibited by 80%. This is not a
generalized inhibition of all sites of autophosphorylation but
of specific sites. Tryptic peptide mapping of labelled receptor
in the presence of antibody revealed that only pY4 and a smaller
peak subsequently denoted as pY5 remain.

Radioactive sequenation of this peak revealed three possible
tyrosines of which two were adjacent to each other and the other
tyrosine was four or five amino acids away. If one examines the
possible autophosphorylation domains of the receptor, it is
clear that the group of tyrosines which cluster around 1150
position resembles the pattern seen in the sequenation data. The
tyrosines are at 1146, 1150 and 1151 positions; according to the
sequence of Rutter's group, they would represent 1158, 1162 and
1163. Thus, the first sites of autophosphorylation exist about
120 amino acids towards the C-terminal from the ATP binding
site.

There is a glutamic acid present between the 1146 tyrosine and
the other two residues allowing V_8 protease digestion. This
site revealed 50% of the radioactivity at 1146 position and
about 50% of the radioactivity at the 1150 and 1151 positions.
From other experiments, it seems that the 1146 tyrosine is
always phosphorylated while either of the 1150 or the 1151
tyrosines may be phosphorylated.

So, is this phosphorylation domain important in triggering the
kinase activity? When one examines substrate phosphorylation
with this partially phosphorylated receptor, it was found that
there is activation of the kinase activity at low substrate
concentrations but no activation at high substrate
concentrations. This type of biphasic activity is typical of a
receptor that is not fully activated (Fig. 4).

Other Domains: There are other potential sites of
phosphorylation which may be important. Antibodies which
specifically react with the 960 domain, fail to recognize any of
the tryptic peptide peaks. Also, substitution of the 960

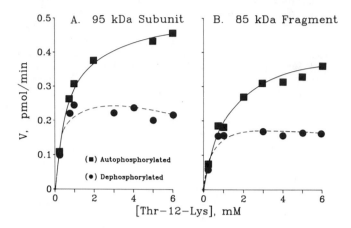

FIGURE 3: Comparison of the 95 kDa subunit and the 85 kDa
fragment with respect to tyrosine kinase activity vs.
synthetic substrate (Thr-12-Lys) concentration. No
significant differences were noted in the dephosphorylated or
the autophosphorylated state.

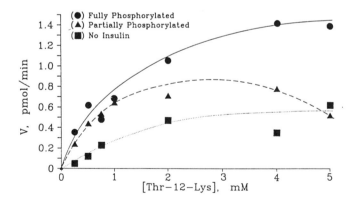

FIGURE 4: Substrate inhibition of receptor kinase activity
during different states of receptor activation using a
partially purified insulin receptor.

tyrosine with phenylalanine did not change the tryptic peptide map of the phosphorylated receptor.

Using antibodies directed against the 1150 domain and radiosequenation techniques, the tryptic peptide peaks, pY1 and pY1a seem to be derived from the 1150 domain and contain 3 phosphotyrosyl residues at positions 1146, 1150 and 1151. When phosphotyrosine antibodies are used to inhibit formation of pY1 and pY1a, larger peaks of pY4 and pY5 are seen, suggesting again that pY4 and pY5 represent the 1150 domain with only two phosphotyrosines. Therefore, when two tyrosines, 1146 and 1150/1151 are phosphorylated, the receptor is only partially active. Full activation requires the tyrosines at 1146 and at both 1150 and 1151 to be phosphorylated. It is not known whether this cascade is via transphosphorylation between β-subunits or via phosphorylation within a single β-subunit.

Intact Cells: In intact cells, the insulin receptor is in a different environment and the autophosphorylation sites are slightly different (Fig. 2) (12). pY4 is the major peak observed and in addition to the previously noted peaks which are less abundant here, there are two other peaks, pS and pT which correspond to the phosphoserine site and the phosphothreonine site. pY4 corresponds to the 1150 domain, the first site of autophosphorylation. pY1 and pY1a peaks are very minor peaks and this is consistent with this domain as being a minor site in the intact cell during the first minute of insulin action. The receptor seems only partially activated in intact cells at this early point (Fig. 5).

Another difference between the phosphorylation of the isolated receptor and the receptor in intact cells is that in the basal state, a major site of serine phosphorylation is observed in intact cells. Data from our laboratory as well as others' (2,5,10) have suggested that this is a result of protein kinase C activity. When one stimulates cells with a phorbol ester, TPA, serine phosphorylation of the receptor is stimulated and subsequent tyrosine phosphorylation of the receptor is inhibited (Fig. 6). The insulin receptor isolated from TPA treated cells has about 50% reduction in its tyrosine kinase activity.

SUMMARY

The insulin receptor contains three separate domains of tyrosine phosphorylation (Fig. 7) in the β-subunit all of which are stimulated by insulin binding to the α-subunit. Autophosphorylation of the receptor has also been thought to initiate the cascade of kinase activity. Activation of the kinase activity occurs over several minutes and is slower than the rapid actions of insulin. We observed that the first site

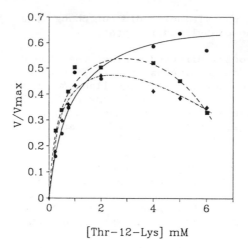

FIGURE 5: The kinase activity of the insulin stimulated insulin
receptor autophosphorylated in vitro or in vivo. The
activities of the fully phosphorylated receptor (circles), the
partially phosphorylated receptor in the presence of
antiphosphotyrosine antibody (diamonds) and the in vivo
labelled receptor (squares) are depicted by plotting v/V_{max}
against substrate concentration.

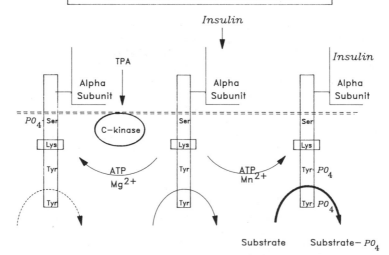

FIGURE 6: Regulation of the insulin receptor by multisite
phosphorylation. A schematic representation of activation of
the insulin receptor kinase by autophosphorylation and
inhibition by possible serine phosphorylation by protein
kinase C.

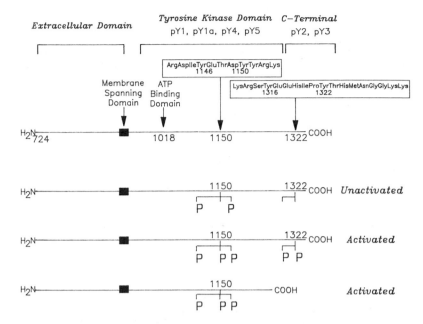

FIGURE 7:   Linear model of the insulin receptor.   Important
   domains are summarized.   The receptor must have a triply
   phosphorylated 1150 domain to be fully active as a tyrosine
   kinase.   The C-terminal, though phosphorylated, does not seem
   to play a role in activation of the kinase.

of autophosphorylation with two phosphotyrosines in the 1150
domain is not sufficient for full kinase activity. The
C-terminal domain containing the 1316 and 1322 tyrosines is
autophosphorylated but its absence does not affect the tyrosine
kinase activity of the receptor. The autophosphorylation domain
containing the 953 and 960 tyrosines is not an important domain
We find that the triply phosphorylated 1150 domain is essential
for full kinase activity. Our conclusion is supported by the
data of Ellis et al (4) who studied the kinase activity of an
insulin receptor mutated at the 1150 and 1151 sites. Thus
insulin receptor phosphorylation begins by phosphorylation of
1146 tyrosine and of either 1150 or 1151 tyrosine and progresses
to phosphorylation of the third tyrosine resulting in full
kinase activity.

   During the early time points of insulin action in intact
cells, the partially activated receptor is observed instead of
the fully activated form. In intact cells, serine
phosphorylation of the insulin receptor, possibly via protein
kinase C may regulate tyrosine autophosphorylation as well as
exogenous protein tyrosine kinase activity.

ACKNOWLEDGEMENT

The authors wish to thank Ms. Terri-Lyn Bellman for her excellent secretarial assistance in the preparation of this manuscript.

REFERENCES

1. Avruch,J., Nemenoff, R.A., Blackshear, P.J., Pierce, M.W. and Osathanondh, R.: (1982) J. Biol. Chem. 258:15162-15166.
2. Bollag, G.E., Roth, R.A., Beaudoin, J., Mochly-Rosen, D. and Koshland,Jr., D.E.: (1986) Proc. Natl. Acad. Sci. USA 83:5822-5824.
3. Ebina, Y., Ellis, L., JArnagin, K., Edery, M., Graf, L., Clauser, E., Ou, J.H., Masiarz, F., Kan, Y.W., Goldfine, I.D., Roth, R.A. and Rutter, W.J.: (1985) Cell 40:747-758.
4. Ellis, L., Clauser, E., Morgan, D.O., Edery, M., Roth, R.A. and Rutter, W.J.: (1986) Cell 45:721-732.
5. Jacobs, S., Sahyoun, N.E., Saltiel, A.R. and Cuatrecasas, P.: (1983) Proc. Natl. Acad. Sci. USA 80:6211-6213.
6. Kahn, C.R.: (1985) Annu. Rev. Med. 36:429-451.
7. Kasuga, M., Karlsson, F.A. and Kahn, C.R.: (1982) Science 215:185-187.
8. Pilch, P.F. and Czech, M.P.: (1979) J. Biol. Chem. 254:3375-3381.
9. Rosen, O.M., Herrera, R., Olowe, Y., Petruzelli, M. and Cobb, M.H.: (1983) Proc. Natl. Acad. Sci. USA 80:3237-3240.
10. Takayama, S., White, M.F., Lauris, V. and Kahn, C.R.: (1984) Proc. Natl. Acad. Sci. USA 81:7797-7800.
11. Ullrich, A., Bell, J.R., Chen, E.Y., Herrera, R., Petruzelli, L.M., Dull, T.J., Gray, A.,Coussens, L., Liao, Y.C., Tsubokawa, M., Mason, A., Seeburg, P.H., Grunfeld, C., Rosen, O.M. and Ramachandran, J.: (1985) Nature 313:756-761.
12. White, M.F., Takayama, S. and Kahn, C.R.: (1984) J. Biol. Chem. 260:9470-9475.
13. White, M.F., Haring, H.U., Kasuga, M. and Kahn, C.R.: (1984) J. Biol. Chem. 259:255-264.
14. Yu, K.T. and Czech, M.P.: (1984) J. Biol. Chem. 259:5277-5286.

Insulin Action and Diabetes,
edited by H. Joseph Goren et al.
Raven Press, New York © 1988.

IDENTIFICATION OF THE INSULIN RECEPTOR TYROSINE RESIDUES
AUTOPHOSPHORYLATED IN VITRO AND IN VIVO: RELATIONSHIP
TO RECEPTOR KINASE ACTIVATION

Hans E. Tornqvist[*], J. Ryan Gunsalus and Joseph Avruch

From the Howard Hughes Medical Institute Laboratories,
Harvard Medical School; Medical Services and Diabetes Unit
Massachusetts General Hospital and the Department of Medicine
Harvard Medical School, Boston, MA 02114
*Current Address: Department of Pediatrics
University Hospital, University of Lund,
S-221 85 Lund, Sweden

INTRODUCTION

Regulatory protein phosphorylation is involved at several steps in the sequence of reactions by which insulin reorients cell function (1). The insulin receptor is itself a tyrosine-specific protein kinase (4,11), and abolition of insulin receptor β subunit autophosphorylation in intact cells, whether achieved through expression of cloned insulin receptors whose ATP binding site has been inactivated by mutagenesis (2,3), or through introduction into cells of monoclonal antibodies which inhibit receptor autophosphorylation (6,7), completely blocks insulin action. Thus, insulin-stimulated tyrosine-specific autophosphorylation of the β subunit is a regulatory phosphorylation which is the first intracellular step in insulin action. Two general models can be formulated in regard to the nature of the requirement for receptor autophosphorylation (Fig. 1).

Model 1 envisions signalling mediated entirely through the receptor-catalyzed tyrosine phosphorylation of other proteins; Model 2 envisions signalling mediated through the noncovalent interaction of the autophosphorylated β subunit with one or more "coupling" proteins; receptor catalyzed covalent modification of other proteins is irrelevant.

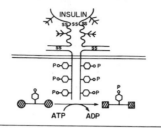

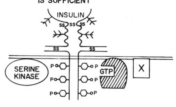

FIG. 1. The Mechanism of Signal Transmission by the Autophosphorylated Insulin Receptor.

These models are not exclusive, but in either instance, autophosphorylation is the initial critical event, inasmuch as the ability of the receptor to phosphorylate other proteins in an insulin-stimulated reaction in vitro is entirely dependent on some component of β subunit tyrosine autophosphorylation (10). In view of the central role of β subunit autophosphorylation in insulin action, we have undertaken a detailed analysis of the molecular anatomy of this reaction; the majority of the multiple tyrosine residues which participate in the insulin-stimulated autophosphorylation of the partially purified human IR in vitro have been identified directly by amino acid sequence analysis (8) and compared to the sites phosphorylated in the intact rat hepatoma cells (9); these prove to be essentially identical. In addition, the relationship of site-specific autophosphorylation to the activation of the tyrosine protein kinase has been defined (10).

Identification of the Insulin Receptor Autophosphorylation Sites (8,9)

Previous studies from our laboratory indicated that in the presence of insulin, an identical extent of overall ^{32}P incorporation into Tyr residues on the β subunit of the partially purified human IR was achieved on incubation with ATP and either manganese or magnesium, and overall Tyr(P) formation

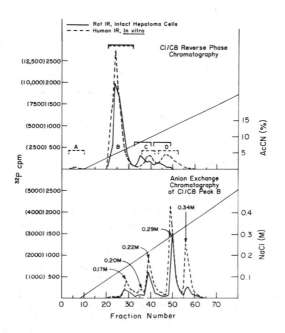

FIG. 2.   Chromatographic   Profiles   of   [^{32}P]Tyr(P)-containing
Tryptic   Peptides   Derived   from   Insulin   Receptor
Autophosphorylated In Vitro and in Intact Cells.

    Immunoaffinity   purified   [^{32}P]Tyr(P)-containing   tryptic
peptides derived from 1) human IR equilibrated with 0.1 μM
insulin and autophosphorylated in vitro (10 mM, Mn^{++}, 0.2 mM
ATP, 1 min at 23°C) to approximately 50°/° of maximal kinase
activation (dashed line), and 2) rat IR autophosphorylated in
intact ^{32}P-labelled hepatoma cells exposed to insulin (1 μM, 5
min, solid line) were separated by C1/C8 reverse-phase
chromatography (upper panel). The major C1/C8 peak (B) was
subjected to anion-exchange chromatography (lower panel).

correlated closely with the extent of activation of the tyrosine
protein   kinase   (5).   To   optimize   recovery   of
[^{32}P]Tyr(P)-containing peptides which serve as phosphorylation
sites, autophosphorylation of the partially purified human
(placental) IR was allowed to proceed in the presence of insulin
and Mn plus [γ-^{32}P]ATP so as to attain a near maximal extent
of kinase activation. The ^{32}P-labelled IR was purified by
immunoaffinity chromatography on antiphosphotyrosine monoclonal
antibodies coupled to Sepharose 4B. All ^{32}P-labelled IR was
recovered in this step, and shown to contain only [^{32}P]Tyr(P)

K<u>III GPLIFVFLFS VVIGSIYLFL</u> RKRQPDGPLG PLYASSNPEY LSASDVFPCS (970)

VYVPDEWEVS REKITLLREL GQGSFGMVYE GNARDIIKGE AETRVAVKTV NESAS (1025)

LRERI EFLNEASVMK GFTCHHVVRL LGVVSKGQPT LVVMELMAHG DLKSYLRSLR (1080)

PEAENNPGRP PPTLQEMINM AAEIADGMAY LNAKKFVHRD LAARNCMVAH DFTVK (1135)

IGDFG MTRDIYETDY YRKGGKGLLP VRWMAPESLK DGVFTTSSDM WSFGVVLWEI (1190)

TSLAEQPYQG LSNEQVLKFV MDGGYLDQPD NCPERVTDLM RMCWQFNPNM RPTFL (1245)

EIVNL LKDDLHPSFP EVSFFHSEEN KAPESEELEM EFEDMENVPL DRSSHCQREE (1300)

AGGRDGGSSL GFKRSYEEHI PYTHMNGGKK NGRILTLPRS NPS (1343)

FIG. 3. Amino Acid sequence of the transmembranous and intracellular portions of the human insulin receptor β subunit.

The single letter code is displayed. The residue number ending each line corresponds to the residue immediately preceeding, and is taken from Ullrich, et al. (11). A space separates every 10 residues. The putative transmembrane segment is underlined by an open rectangle. The 8 intracellular tryptic peptides which contain tyrosine are indicated by a line drawn above, and are numbered (1-8) from the transmembrane region toward the C-terminus. The 13 intracellular tyrosine residues are indicated by arrows.

on phosphoamino acid analysis. ^{32}P-labelled β subunit purified by SDS gel electrophoresis was subjected to exhaustive tryptic digestion. The tryptic peptides containing Tyr(P) were purified by antiphosphotyrosine immunoaffinity chromatography followed by sequential reverse-phase (C1/C8) and anion-exchange chromatography; > 80°/° recovery of ^{32}P was achieved at each step (Fig. 2). On the reverse-phase column, four peaks were generally seen designated A-D (Fig. 2 upper). Peak B always contained 70-80°/° of recovered ^{32}P, and when subjected to anion-exchange chromatography, was resolved into five peaks; two minor peaks eluting at 0.17, 0.20 M NaCl and three major peaks eluting at 0.22, 0.29 and 0.34 M NaCl (Fig. 2, lower). Peak D contains 10-15°/° of recovered ^{32}P and is composed predominantly of a tryptic peptide of M_r 4000-5000 (not shown); all other ^{32}P is recovered in tryptic peptides of M_r < 2000, as analyzed by SDS/urea polyacrylamide gradient gel electrophoresis. Peak A and C were minor and not further characterized.

Identification of the major [^{32}P]Tyr(P) peptides was achieved by gas-phase microsequencing. The partial amino acid sequence obtained was compared to the amino acid sequence deduced from the nucleotide sequence of the intracellular extension of the insulin receptor β subunit (Fig. 3). By this approach, the major components of reverse-phase peak B, which account for at least 60°/° of all [^{32}P]Tyr(P) in the maximally autophosphorylated receptor, were shown to be peptide 8 (SYEEHIPYTHMNGGK; eluting at 0.22 M NaCl on anion-exchange chromatography), and two charge isoforms of peptide 5 (DIYETDYYR, eluting at 0.29 M NaCl and 0.34 M NaCl). These two peptides, 5 and 8, are recovered in roughly equal molar quantities and contain 5 of the 13 intracellular tyrosines on the receptor. The specific tyrosine residues on peptide 5 and 8 which undergo phosphorylation were identified by a combination of solid-phase Edman degradation and subdigestion with Staphylococcus aureus V8 protease, as described in a succeeding presentation; these studies indicated that the ^{32}P-peptide eluting at 0.22 M NaCl is a double phosphorylated form of peptide 8 (Tyr(P) at residue 1316 and 1322), whereas the ^{32}P-peptide eluting at 0.29 M NaCl and 0.34 M NaCl are the double (Tyr(P) at residue 1146 equals that at residue 1150 plus 1151) and triple phosphorylated forms of peptide 5. Peak D, which contains another 10-15°/° of [^{32}P]Tyr(P), was not identified directly, but based on its apparent M_r can only be tryptic peptide 1 and/or 6. We believe that peptide 1 is the more likely candidate, because in examining synthetic peptides corresponding to tryptic peptides 1-8 as substrates for the insulin receptor kinase in vitro, tryptic peptides 1, 5 and 8 are clearly the best substrates, whereas the peptide corresponding to peptide 6 is a poor substrate. These three peptides, i.e. 5, 8 and (probably) 1, encompass at least 75°/° of the [^{32}P]Tyr(P) incorporated in the receptor during autophosphorylation in vitro.

This information is significant only insofar as it reflects the reaction which occurs when insulin is added to intact cells. To determine the sites of "in vivo" receptor autophosphorylation, we treated ^{32}P-labelled rat hepatoma cells (H4-II-E-C3) with supramaximal concentrations of insulin for 5 min and purified the Triton X-100 extracted Tyr(P)-containing proteins by immunoaffinity chromatography on columns of monoclonal antiphosphotyrosine antibodies coupled to Sepharose 4B. As seen in Fig. 4, only two major insulin-stimulated [^{32}P]Tyr(P)-containing proteins are found in the hapten eluate, M_r 95,000 and 180,000. The M_r 95,000 protein is the β subunit of the insulin receptor, as indicated by its immunoprecipitation by several antireceptor antisera, including two sera raised against synthetic peptides corresponding to the major autophosphorylated domains on human IR, i.e. tryptic peptides 5 and 8. The M_r 180,000 protein, by contrast, is unreactive with all anti-insulin receptor antisera. These same two proteins are also detected by immune blotting of nonradioactive extracts from control- and

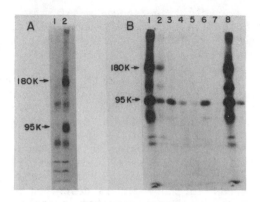

FIG. 4. A: Rat Hepatoma Cell [^{32}P]Tyr(P)-containing Proteins Adsorbed by Monoclonal Antiphosphotyrosine antibodies.

^{32}P-labelled rat hepatoma cells (H4-II-E-C3) were exposed to diluent (lane 1) or insulin (lane 2, 1 μM) for 5 min, solubilized and adsorbed to columns of monoclonal antiphosphotyrosine antibody 1G2 (9). After extensive washing, [^{32}P]Tyr(P)-containing proteins were selectively eluted with 40 mM phenyl phosphate. The two major insulin-stimulated ^{32}P-labelled proteins at M_r 180,000 and 95,000 were both shown to contain [^{32}P]Tyr(P) by two-dimensional thin-layer electrophoresis after total hydrolysis.

B: Immunoprecipitation of ^{32}P-labelled Rat Insulin Receptor.

The eluate depicted in lane A2 above (represented in B at 1 x in lanes 1 and 8 and 0.1 x in lane 2) was subjected to immunoprecipitation with: lane 3 - rabbit antisera versus the synthetic peptide RDIYETDYYRK corresponding to residues 1143-1153 of the human IR (this sequence is identical in the rat IR); lane 4 - rabbit antisera versus the synthetic peptide KRSYEEHIPY, corresponding to residues 1313-1322 of the human IR (the homologous segment in rat IR has the sequence KRTYDEHIPY); lane 5 - rabbit antisera to peptide KTRPEDFRD, corresponding to residues 40-48 in human IR (sequence of homologous segment in rat IR is unknown); lane 6 - human antiserum (B2) reactive with the human IR; lane 7 - normal rabbit serum. After overnight incubation at 4°C, the immune complexes were harvested with pansorbin, washed and analyzed by autoradiography after SDS PAGE; it is reprinted from Ref. 9.

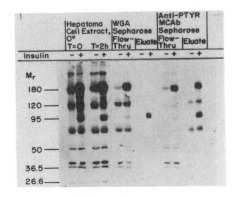

FIG. 5. Immunoblot of Control and Insulin-treated Rat Hepatoma Cell Proteins with Polyclonal Antiphosphotyrosine Antibodies.

Rat hepatoma cells were exposed to insulin (1 μM) or diluent for 5 min, and extracted as in Ref. 9. Aliquots of the (nonradioactive) extract were subjected to SDS-PAGE immediately (lanes 1 and 2) or after 2 hrs at 0°C (lanes 3 and 4); another aliquot was adsorbed to wheat-germ agglutinin Sepharose, and the flow-through (lanes 5 and 6) and N-acetylglucosamine eluate (lanes 7 and 8) fractions subjected to SDS-PAGE (lanes 7 and 8); a last aliquot was adsorbed to a column of monoclonal antiphosphotyrosine antibody 1G2 (as in Fig. 4A), and the flow-through lanes 9 and 10)and phenylphosphate eluates (lanes 11 and 12) subjected to SDS-PAGE. The proteins were transferred to nitrocellulose, exposed to a polyclonal antiphosphotyrosine antibody (9) and the immunoreactive bands identified by binding of ^{125}I-protein A; it is reprinted from Ref. 9.

insulin-treated hepatoma cells, using an independently generated polyclonal antiphosphotyrosine antibody. This reagent also permits an examination of the proteins which flow-through the monoclonal antibody column: as evident in Fig. 5, the Tyr(P)-containing M_r 95,000 β subunit is entirely retained by the monoclonal antibody column and recovered in the phenylphosphate eluate. Conversely, the Tyr(P)-containing M_r 180,000 protein is only partially retained on the column[a].

[a]Little is known about this M_r 180,000 protein, which was first detected by White, et al (12). We find that it is extractable from cells by homogenization in buffers lacking detergent, or containing low concentrations of digitonin sufficient to lyse the cell, but insufficient to extract the insulin receptor or mitochondrial enzymes. It is not bound to lectin columns, and can occasionally be resolved into two closely spaced bands on SDS-PAGE. A report providing more extensive characterization of this putative substrate for the IR kinase is in preparation.

The high recovery of Tyr(P)-containing M_r 95,000 β subunit in this eluate provided a suitably representative starting material for identification of IR tryptic peptides which contain [^{32}P]Tyr(P); this was accomplished by the approach applied successfully to the human IR phosphorylated in vitro, as described above. The ^{32}P-labelled M_r 95,000 β subunit was eluted from SDS gels and digested to completion with trypsin. The [^{32}]Tyr(P) tryptic peptides were isolated by antiphosphotyrosine immunoaffinity chromatography; phosphoamino acid analysis demonstrated that all [^{32}P]Tyr(P)-containing peptides are bound to the column. The nonadsorbed fraction, which contains about 50°/° of applied ^{32}P, contains no detectable [^{32}P]Tyr(P). Moreover, all ^{32}P in the peptides eluted from the antiphosphotyrosine antibody column was [^{32}P]Tyr(P); no [^{32}P]Ser(P) or [^{32}P]Thr(P) is detectable in the [^{32}P]Tyr(P)-containing tryptic peptides. The [^{32}P]Tyr(P)-tryptic peptides were then separated by sequential reverse-phase (C1/C8) and anion-exchange (Mono Q) chromatography, as before (Fig. 2). The profiles of ^{32}P observed (which reflect only [^{32}P]Tyr(P)) were essentially identical to those obtained from digests of human IR autophosphorylated in vitro, including an M_r 4000-5000 as the principal component of C1/C8 peak D, as judged by SDS/urea PAGE. The major peaks of rat IR [^{32}P]Tyr(P)-peptide were analyzed by gas-phase microsequencing, solid-phase Edman degradation and subdigestion with Staphylococcus aureus V8 protease; the partial amino acid sequence obtained was compared to the amino acid sequence of the intracellular extension of the rat IR β subunit (deduced from genomic sequence, determined by R.E. Lewis, M.P. Czech and M.A. Tepper and communicated to us prior to publication). The results showed that 90°/° of all β subunit [^{32}P]Tyr(P) resides on three tryptic peptides: 1) 50-60°/° is on the peptide, DIYETDYYR, which is recovered mainly as the double phosphorylated species (Tyr(P) at residue 3 from the aminoterminus = Tyr(P) at residues 7 plus 8) with 10-15°/° as the triple phosphorylated species. 2) A second peptide has the sequence TYDEHIPYTHMNGGK, contains about 20-30°/° of β subunit [^{32}P]Tyr(P) and is located near the carboxyterminus; it is recovered in the double phosphorylated form. 3) Lastly, approximately 10°/° of β subunit [^{32}P]Tyr(P) is recovered on the M_r 4000-5000 tryptic peptide, which we presume to be homologous to the peptide of corresponding size detected in digests of the human IR autophosphorylated in vitro.

Thus, the tyrosine residues autophosphorylated on the rat IR in intact hepatoma cells exposed to a supramaximal concentration of insulin (1.0 μM) for 5 min are identical to those undergoing phosphorylation on the partially purified human IR incubated with insulin (0.1 μM), Mn^{++} (10 mM), ATP (200 μM): at least 6 of the 13 tyrosines on the intracellular extension of the receptor participate in this reaction. These residues in vivo and in vitro, are distributed on three domains in clusters of closely spaced Tyr(P): a cluster of Tyr(P) is found on a peptide segment (DIYETDYYR) located in the "tyrosine kinase domain" which contains 2 or 3 Tyr(P) within 6 amino acids. This segment is homologous to the major in vitro autophosphorylation site of Rous sarcoma virus-transforming antigen. A second cluster of two Tyr(P) is located near the carboxyterminus, in a region where the insulin receptor is least similar in amino acid sequence to other tyrosine kinase receptors, including the IGF-1 receptor. A third phosphorylated region corresponds to human IR tryptic peptides 1 and/or 6 (probably 1) and contains at least one (potentially up to 3) Tyr(P) residues.

Relationship of Site-specific β Subunit Autophosphorylation to Activation of Receptor Tyrosine Kinase (10)

The regulation of the insulin receptor kinase activity by insulin and intramolecular autophosphorylation exhibits several features which are unique among ligand-activated protein kinases. The most important feature is that the ability of the ligand, insulin, to activate the protein kinase activity, is completely dependent on prior β subunit tyrosine autophosphorylation. This is illustrated by the experiment shown in Fig. 6: insulin receptor is incubated with Mn alone or MnATP, and at intervals the autophosphorylation is terminated by addition of excess EGTA. The receptor kinase can then be assayed by dilution and addition of MgATP and histone 2b. At concentrations of MgATP well below K_m, high concentrations of histone 2b and other model protein/peptide substrates inhibit β subunit autophosphorylation and kinase activation (5). Consequently, the histone 2b tyrosine kinase activity of the receptor can be measured under conditions, such that further receptor autophosphorylation during the assay per se is drastically or completely inhibited. In such an assay, insulin at saturating concentrations (1 μM) does not stimulate histone kinase activity at all unless preincubation with MnATP has occurred. Conversely, preincubation with MnATP in the absence of insulin does permit kinase activation. The event critical for activation is the provision of metal/ATP so as to permit β subunit tyrosine autophosphorylation[b]. Preincubation with MnATP does not merely augment an activation by insulin, but is required absolutely for insulin stimulation of receptor kinase to occur. The sole function of insulin is to stimulate β subunit autophosphorylation.

[b]In the presence of insulin, preincubation with MgATP at saturating concentrations will activate receptor kinase to the same extent as saturating MnATP, but Mn or Mg plus AMPPCP produces no activation.

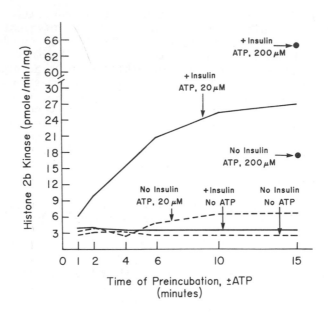

FIG. 6. Insulin Activation of Receptor Kinase is Completely Dependent on Autophosphorylation.

Partially purified human placental insulin receptor was preincubated ± insulin (1 μM, 30 min, 23°C). At t=0 min, Mn (10 mM) or Mn (10 mM) + ATP (20 μM) was added. At t=1, 2, 4, 6, 10 and 15 min, aliquots were removed into excess EGTA (15 mM). Two other aliquots of receptor (± insulin) were incubated with 200 μM ATP for 15 min prior to addition of EGTA. Histone 2b tyrosine kinase in each sample was assayed in the presence of histone 2b (5.5 mg/ml), Mg (10 mM) and [^{32}P-γ]ATP (20 μM, 40 cpm/fmol). Dilution of the first incubation was such that carryover of ATP into the second incubation (kinase assay) was always < 2 μM. Under these conditions, which prevent intra-assay autophosphorylation, insulin is without effect on kinase activity unless ATP was present in the preincubation.

A further insight into the nature of kinase activation was obtained by utilizing antiphosphotyrosine monoclonal antibodies: insulin receptor kinase was brought to increasing degrees of activation, in the presence of insulin, by incubation with MnATP for various times and quench with EGTA. Adsorption of these partially activated mixtures to antiphosphotyrosine monoclonal antibodies removed all of the ^{32}P-labelled insulin receptor and all of the insulin-activated component of histone 2b tyrosine kinase; the nonadsorbed fraction exhibited no "stimulated" kinase activity. However the absence of activated kinase and ^{32}P-labelled insulin receptor in this fraction did not reflect the absence of residual receptors; further incubation of the nonadsorbed fraction with MgATP generated substantial kinase activity, approaching that expected based on the percent of receptor kinase which remained unactivated in the first autophosphorylation reaction. This result not only provides further evidence for the obligatory relationship between β subunit tyrosine autophosphorylation and kinase activation, but illustrates the exceptionally concerted nature of the activation process in the presence of insulin: partially autophosphorylated, partially activated receptor preparations are actually mixtures of receptors which are unphosphorylated and unactivated, together with receptors that are highly phosphorylated and completely or nearly completely activated.

In the presence of insulin, overall β subunit ^{32}P incorporation tracks closely with the extent of kinase activation, up to about 90°/° of maximal kinase (5,8). The peptide mapping techniques developed for analysis of the fully phosphorylated receptor (described above), were applied to receptor preparations activated in the presence of insulin over the entire range of histone 2b kinase activity. Not unexpectedly, the highly concerted character of the kinase activation is mirrored by the concerted nature of the autophosphorylation. The tryptic maps of receptors autophosphorylated so as to achieve from 2°/° to 90°/° of maximal kinase activity are indistinguishable: phosphorylation on all three domains (the M_r 4000 tryptic peptide, the tryptic peptide containing Tyr 1146/1150/1151, and the carboxyterminal tryptic peptide) is detected at all extents of autophosphorylation. More remarkable yet is the detection of double and triple phosphorylated peptide segments in substantial proportions, even at activations of under 5°/°. Thus autophosphorylation is almost an "all or none" transition, proceeding in a nearly concurrent fashion on several β subunit domains, and leading to kinase activation.

Does this concerted multisite phosphorylation mean that phosphorylation of all domains is equally important to kinase activation? Insight on this point was gained by examining the correlation between autophosphorylation and kinase activation in the absence and presence of insulin. Insulin dramatically stimulates the initial rate of overall β subunit autophosphorylation under all conditions, but at saturating metal/ATP, overall ^{32}P incorporation in the absence of insulin can proceed to 30-50°/° of the extent observed in the presence of insulin[c]. Activation of kinase is observed as a concomitant of this insulin-independent (basal) autophosphorylation, but autophosphorylation in the absence of insulin is considerably less productive of kinase activation, i.e. less overall β subunit phosphorylation produces a higher kinase activity in the presence of insulin. This is not due to the phosphorylation of unique sites in the presence of insulin; the tryptic maps of insulin receptor autophosphorylated in the presence and absence of insulin are qualitatively similar, and no "new" peaks are observed in the presence of insulin. Insulin stimulates phosphorylation of all domains, especially at early times. Nevertheless, the difference in the efficiency of autophosphorylation in producing kinase activation, depending on the presence or absence of insulin, permits qualitative comparisons of the pattern of site-specific autophosphorylation under conditions of comparable overall β subunit ^{32}P incorporation, but very different kinase activity or comparable kinase activity achieved at different overall ^{32}P incorporation. In all such comparisons, ^{32}P incorporation into the tryptic peptide containing Tyr 1146/1150/1151 tracks very closely with kinase activity; incorporation into the M_r 4000 tryptic peptide correlates nearly as well. By contrast, ^{32}P incorporation into the tryptic peptide from the carboxyterminus, which contains Tyr(P) at 1316 and 1322, is frequently dissociated from extent of kinase activation. These observations lead us to conclude that phosphorylation of the former two domains is critical for the initiation and/or maintenance of kinase activation, whereas phosphorylation of the carboxyterminal Tyr residues is not. Phosphorylation of this region may be irrelevant to receptor function, but more likely, is critical for some function unrelated to kinase activation per se, e.g. signalling, internalization, clustering, etc.

In conclusion, insulin-stimulated β subunit autophosphorylation is the first intracellular reaction in the sequence of steps by which insulin changes cell function. We have identified the tyrosine residues which participate in this reaction both in vitro and in intact cells. In both situations, insulin stimulates the phosphorylation of at least 6 of 13 tyrosine residues situated on the intracellular extension of the β subunit. These are distributed as clusters on three β subunit

---

[c] In intact cells, β subunit tyrosine phosphorylation is not detectable in the absence of insulin. Although this may simply signify that the activity of cellular phosphotyrosine phosphatases are in excess of the rate of basal receptor autophosphorylation, it is also possible that basal autophosphorylation of the receptor in the cell is totally inhibited, and undergoes a partial "disinhibition" as a consequence of solubilization from the membrane or enzyme purification.

domains: an M_r 4000 tryptic peptide, presumed to be amino acid residues 944-971, just inside the membrane; a second domain in the tyrosine kinase region encompassing the Tyr 1146, 1150, 1151, and which is recovered predominantly in a double and triple phosphorylated state; a segment containing two Tyr(P) at residues 1316 and 1322, near the carboxyterminus. β subunit autophosphorylation in vitro proceeds in a highly concerted fashion in the presence and absence of insulin, with phosphorylation of multiple Tyr residues on all three domains proceeding in a nearly concurrent fashion, and kinase activation occurring with similar abruptness. The ability of insulin to cause kinase activation is completely dependent on prior β subunit autophosphorylation, and phosphorylation of the Tyr residues at 1146/1150/1151, and on the M_r 4000 tryptic peptide track closely with the extent of kinase activation. Phosphorylation of the tyrosines in the carboxyterminal domain, although substantially stimulated by insulin, is frequently dissociated from the concomitant kinase activity in vitro, and probably subserves a function in vivo other than activation of the kinase.

REFERENCES

1. Avruch, J., Nemenoff, R.A., Pierce, M.W., Kwok, Y.C., and Blackshear, P.J. (1985): In: Molecular Basis of Insulin Action. edited by M.P. Czech, pp. 263-295. Plenum Press, New York.
2. Chou, C.K., Dull, T.J., Russell, D.S., Gherzi, R., Lebwohl, D., Ullrich, A., and Rosen, O.M. (1987): J. Biol. Chem., 267:1842-1847.
3. Ebina, Y., Araki, E., Tanra, M., Shumada, F., Mori, M., Fraik, C.S., Siddle, K., Pierce, S.B., Roth, R.A., and Rutter, W.J. (1987): Proc. Natl. Acad. Sci. USA, 84, 704-708.
4. Ebina, Y., Ellis, L., Jarnagin, K., Edery, M., Graf, L., Clauser, E., Ou, J-H., Marsiaz, F., Kan, Y.W., Goldfine, D., Roth, R.A., and Rutter, W.J. (1985): Cell, 40:747-748.
5. Kwok, Y.C., Nemenoff, R.A., Powers, A.C., and Avruch, J. (1986): Arch. Biochem. Biophys., 244:102-113.
6. Morgan, D.O., Lisa, H.O., Korn, L.J., and Roth, R.A. (1986): Proc. Natl. Acad. Sci. USA, 83:329-332.
7. Morgan, D.O., and Roth, R.A. (1987): Proc. Natl. Acad. Sci. USA, 84:41-45.
8. Tornqvist, H.E., Pierce, M.W., Frackelton, A.R., Nemenoff, R.A., and Avruch, J. (1987): J. Biol. Chem., 262:10212-10219.
9. Tornqvist, H.E., Gunsalus, J.R., Nemenoff, R.A., Frackelton, A.R., Pierce, M.W., and Avruch, J. (1988): J. Biol. Chem., in press.
10. Tornqvist, H.E., and Avruch, (1987); submitted.
11. Ullrich, A., Bell, J.R., Chen, E.-Y., Herrera, R., Petruzelli, L.M., Dull, T.J., Gray, A., Coussens, L., Liao, Y.-C., Tsubokawa, M., Mason, A., Seeburg, P.H., Grunfield, C., Rosen, O.M., and Ramachandran, J. (1985): Nature, 313:756-761.
12. White, M.F., Maron, R., and Kahn, C.R. (1985): Nature, 318:183-186.

Insulin Action and Diabetes,
edited by H. Joseph Goren et al.
Raven Press, New York © 1988.

IDENTIFICATION OF [^{32}P]Tyr(P) ON MULTIPLE PHOSPHORYLATED
PEPTIDES FROM THE INSULIN RECEPTOR β SUBUNIT

Hans E. Tornqvist*, David Hirshfield and Joseph Avruch

From the Howard Hughes Medical Institute Laboratories,
Harvard Medical School; Medical Services and Diabetes Unit
Massachusetts General Hospital and the Department of Medicine
Harvard Medical School, Boston, MA 02114
*Current Address: Department of Pediatrics
University Hospital, University of Lund,
S-221 85 Lund, Sweden

As described in a previous presentation, the insulin
receptor β subunit catalyzes the intramolecular phosphorylation
of multiple tyrosine residues in the course of the
autophosphorylation reaction. Moreover, these Tyr(P) prove to
be distributed in clusters so that a single tryptic peptide
containing 2 or 3 tyrosines may be recovered in multiple charge
isomers, as a result of the differential phosphorylation of one
or more of these Tyr. This presentation describes the use of
solid-phase Edman degradation together with subdigestion with
Staphylococcal V8 protease to establish the presence of Tyr(P)
at specific residues on ^{32}P-labelled tryptic peptides derived
from insulin receptor β subunit.

Identification of Tyr(P) in Amino Acid Sequence Analysis

We examined the behavior of authentic Tyr(P) in the manual
Edman reaction to determine the yield of ATZ-Tyr(P) and PTH
Tyr(P), as well as the extent of hydrolysis of the phosphate
group under conditions of coupling, conversion and cleavage
(i.e. exposure to anhydrous TFA). Thin-layer electrophoresis on
cellulose plates at pH 1.9 was found to be the most convenient
way to separate Tyr, Tyr(P), ATZ- and PTH Tyr(P) and P$_i$; these
species were detected by fluorescence quenching or comigration
with ^{32}P$_i$. Tyr(P) was not hydrolyzed during coupling and
was stable under the conditions of acid cleavage. PTH Tyr(P)
was however essentially completely insoluble in the solvents

usually employed for extraction of PTH amino acids (e.g. butyl chloride, ethylacetate, etc.), but quite soluble in water; thus, efficient extraction of PTH Tyr(P) required solvents that would produce unacceptly high loss of peptide in conventional liquid or gas-phase amino acid sequencing. The low extrability of PTH Tyr(P) is probably a major factor in the very poor recovery of PTH Tyr(P) in these procedures. Liquid-phase sequencing should be suitable for detection of the [^{32}P]Tyr(P) closest to the NH$_2$ terminus, as with [^{32}P]Ser(P). However, with both Ser(P) and Tyr(P), ^{32}P trails extensively into later cycles, and prevents unambiguous identification of a second phosphoamino acid located further from the N-terminus, unless it contains much more ^{32}P than the first. To overcome the difficulty posed by the similar solubility of ^{32}P-peptide and [^{32}P]Tyr(P), ^{32}P-peptides were coupled via their free carboxyl groups to NH$_2$ derivatized solid supports, using a water soluble carbodiimide (1). This reaction proceeds with high (40-100°/°) efficiency, as long as competing carboxyl groups (e.g. TFA) and primary and secondary amines are completely removed from the sample and solutions prior to coupling. Solid-phase Edman degradation permits extensive washing of the covalently bound peptide with aqueous solvent after each cleavage, and reasonably efficient recovery of ^{32}P. Total recovery of ^{32}P was usually 30-50°/° of ^{32}P-cpm coupled, which we infer to reflect initial yield of the Edman reaction. Coupling via peptide carboxyl groups has the potential however for introducing a new artifact: if ^{32}P-peptide is coupled exclusively through one or more side chain carboxyls, then Edman degradation of this acidic residue will release the remaining undegraded ^{32}P-peptide on acid cleavage; given the frequent occurrence of acidic residues aminoterminal to Tyr(P), this situation could be encountered commonly. Measurement of total ^{32}P in the cleavage washes may therefore be misleading in regard to the presence of PTH[^{32}P]Tyr(P), and direct identification of ^{32}P as PTH[^{32}P]Tyr(P), ^{32}P$_i$ or ^{32}P-peptide, as achieved via thin-layer electrophoresis at pH 1.9 (Fig. 1) is preferable.

By this approach, the major IR [^{32}P]Tyr(P)-containing peptides (first separated by sequential immunoaffinity and reverse-phase chromatography), which elute at 0.22 M, 0.29 M and 0.34 M NaCl on anion-exchange chromatography, can be identified confidently based solely on the release of [^{32}P]Tyr(P) during Edman degradation. The presence of Tyr(P) at cycle 2 in the 0.22 M NaCl peak is compatible with only two of the Tyr-containing β subunit tryptic peptides predicted from the cDNA sequence (SYEEHIPYTHMNGGK - peptide 8, or SYLR - peptide 3); the presence of [^{32}P]Tyr(P) at cycle 8 as well is compatible only with peptide 8. Gas-phase microsequencing of the 0.22 M peptide yielded partial sequence confirming the presence of peptide 8 (1). The presence of Tyr(P) at cycle 3

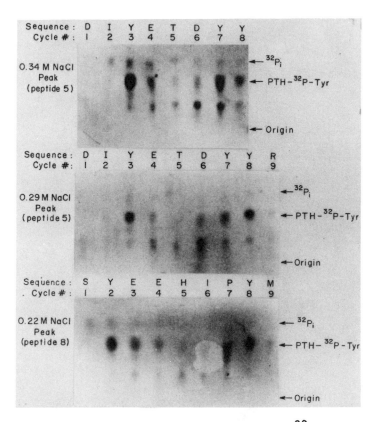

FIG. 1.   Solid-phase Edman Degradation of ^{32}P-labelled IR Tryptic Peptides: Detection of PTH[^{32}P]Tyr(P) by TLE.

The [^{32}P]Tyr(P)-containing tryptic peptides, derived from human IR autophosphorylated in vitro, were separated by anion-exchange chromatography.   The peaks eluting at 0.34 M, 0.29 M and 0.22 M NaCl were coupled via their free carboxyl groups to arylamino-derivatized glass beads, and subjected to manual Edman degradation.   After each TFA cleavage, the beads were washed with pyridine·HCl.   The washes were combined, dried, redissolved in H$_2$O, and a constant aliquot subjected to thin-layer electrophoresis at pH 1.9.   The autoradiograph is shown; it is has been modified from Ref. 1.

for the 0.29 M and 0.34 M NaCl peaks is diagnostic of the IR peptide DIYETDYYR; partial amino acid sequence obtained by gas-phase microsequencing confirmed this identification (1).

The recovery of ^{32}P through the first 4-5 cycles of the solid-phase sequencing is very clearcut; however, a progressive fall in yield accompanied by (and in part, due to) the

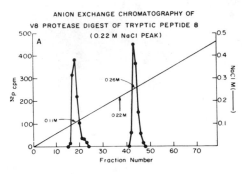

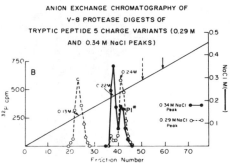

FIG. 2. Staphylococcus aureus V8 Protease Digestion of IR [32P]Tyr(P)-containing Tryptic Peptides.

The IR [32]Tyr(P)-containing tryptic peptides which elute on anion-exchange chromatography at 0.22 M NaCl (upper: panel A), 0.29 M NaCl and 0.34 M NaCl (lower: panel B) were subjected to digestion with Staphylocccus aureus V8 protease (20 µg/ml in ammonium bicarbonate, 50 mM, pH 7.8) for 1 hr at 37°C. The digests were analyzed by anion-exchange chromatography under the conditions originally employed for separation of the undigested parent peptide; the elution position of the undigested peptide is indicated by vertical arrows; modified from Ref. 1.

concomitant release of 32P-peptide renders the quantitative interpretation of total 32P-cpm ambiguous at later cycles. Thin-layer electrophoresis of the cleavage products derived from the 0.22 M NaCl peptide establishes the presence of Tyr(P) at cycle 8, but not the amount. The ambiguity arising from falling yield and carryover is particularly evident with the 0.29 and 0.34 M NaCl 32P-peptides; these two peaks, which both have the primary sequence DIYETDYYR, each appear to contain [32P]Tyr(P) at both of the adjacent tyrosines (residues 7 and 8 from the peptide NH$_2$ terminus). A quantitative estimate is not possible, however, based on the data derived from solid-phase sequencing.

Staphylococcus aureus V8 Protease Subdigestions

The ambiguity regarding the quantitative distribution of Tyr(P) in these multiply phosphorylated peptides is largely resolved by subdigestion of the tryptic peptides with Staphylococcus aureus V8 protease. The peptide eluting at 0.22 M NaCl, shown by solid-phase Edman degradation to be phosphorylated at the tyrosine residues 2 (Tyr 1316) and 8 (Tyr 1322), could be a mixture of two monophosphorylated peptides or a single diphosphorylated peptide. Cleavage with V8 protease C-terminal to the Glu at cycle 3 and/or 4 from the NH$_2$-terminus should give two ^{32}P-peaks on anion-exchange chromatography: a single diphosphorylated peptide will yield two peaks which contain equal amounts of ^{32}P, whereas a mixture of monophosphorylated peptides will be digested into two new peaks which contain ^{32}P in any ratio. The result (Fig. 2A) shows that the 0.22 M peak is cleaved by V8 protease into two new ^{32}P-peptides, which contain equal amounts of ^{32}P, strongly indicative of a double phosphorylated segment (or the formal but unlikely possibility of an equal mixture of monophosphorylated peptides).

Staphylococcus aureus V8 digestion was applied to the 0.29 M and 0.34 M NaCl charge isomers of the peptide DIYETDYYR (Fig. 2B). Both charge forms of this peptide are cleaved completely into two new ^{32}P-peptides; this confirms that both the 0.29 M and 0.34 M NaCl peptides are phosphorylated on Tyr 1146 and 1150 and/or 1151. The more anionic (0.34 M) peptide is cleaved into fragments which contain ^{32}P in a ratio of 2:1, indicating that all three Tyr are phosphorylated. The less anionic version (i.e. the 0.29 M NaCl peptide) is cleaved into two fragments containing equal amounts of ^{32}P. One V8 fragment (eluting at 0.24 M NaCl - Fig. 2B) of the 0.29 M NaCl peptide comigrates with one of the V8 fragments derived from the 0.34 M NaCl peptide; this fragment probably corresponds to the phosphorylated form of DIYE. The second V8 fragment from the 0.29 M peptide elutes earlier (at 0.13 M NaCl) than the corresponding V8 fragment from the 0.34 M NaCl peptide, and is the monophosphorylated form of the peptide TDYYR. Inasmuchas solid-phase Edman degradation demonstrated PTH[^{32}P]Tyr(P) at both residue 7 and 8 from the NH$_2$ terminus of the 0.29 M NaCl peptide with slightly more at cycle 8, then the 0.29 M NaCl peptide is most likely a mixture of two versions of double phosphorylated DIYETDYYR: one with Tyr(P) at residue 3 and 7 and the other with Tyr(P) at residue 3 and 8. The double phosphorylated variety with Tyr(P) at residue 7 and 8 is not present, as this would have generated a third V8 fragment, coeluting with the predominant ^{32}P-labelled V8 fragment of the

0.34 $\underline{M}$ NaCl peptide. Finally, the V8 fragments were themselves coupled to solid supports, and the assignments of Tyr(P) were verified by manual Edman degradation. The data presented above relates to ^{32}P-labelled peptides derived from human IR utophosphorylated in vitro (1). Virtually identical results were obtained with [^{32}P]Tyr(P)-containing tryptic peptides derived from rat IR autophosphorylated in intact hepatoma cells exposed to insulin (2).

In conclusion, the Tyr(P) autophosphorylation sites on the IR are clustered on several short peptides; the peptides were identified by comparison of partial gas-phase amino acid sequence to cDNA sequence. Assignment of [^{32}P]Tyr(P) to specific residues has been accomplished with high certainty by the combined application of solid-phase Edman degradation and subdigestion with Staphylococcus aureus V8 protease.

REFERENCES

1. Tornqvist, H.E., Pierce, M.W., Frackelton, A.R., Nemenoff, R.A., and Avruch, J. (1987): J. Biol. Chem., 262:10212-10219.
2. Tornqvist, H.E., Gunsalus, J.R., Nemenoff, R.A., Frackelton, A.R., Pierce, M.W., and Avruch, J. (1988): J. Biol. Chem., in press.

Insulin Action and Diabetes,
edited by H. Joseph Goren et al.
Raven Press, New York © 1988.

REGULATION OF LIGAND BINDING AND KINASE ACTIVATION IN

ISOLATED INSULIN AND EGF RECEPTORS

Paul F. Pilch, Marianne Boni-Schnetzler and Stephen
Waugh

Department of Biochemistry
Boston University School of Medicine
80 E. Concord St.
Boston, MA   02118

I would like to thank Joe Goren and the organizers
for inviting me to speak here, and I would like to
credit my collaborators, Drs. Marianne Boni-Schnetzler
and Stephen Waugh who are in a large part responsible
for the data I am going to show.
This is my particular version of the insulin
receptor tetrameric structure (Figure 1) which I
usually refer to as a functional dimer because the
receptor is translated as a single, covalently-linked
polyprotein and two such translation products are
disulfide-linked prior to cleavage into individual
alpha and beta subunits. The disulphides which keep
each alpha-beta linked together are virtually un-
reducible, or chemically unreactive for all but de-
naturing conditions, whereas those in the middle can
be reduced and serve to link two identical receptor
halves. So each half of the receptor, as it sits in
the cell surface, has a binding domain and a tyrosine
kinase domain and the overall stoichiometry is two
potential binding sites and two tyrosine kinase
domains per intact insulin receptor. The questions we
want to ask are: 1. How does this structure relate to
function? 2. Are two binding sites used per tetramer
or is there one occupied binding site per tetramer? 3.
How do two halves interact to stimulate kinase
activity? The latter is a particularly interesting
question because there is only a single helical region
that spans the membrane, and from principles of
protein chemistry, it is difficult to imagine how
insulin would bind to this domain of the receptor and

transduce a signal through a rigid helical region.
The model we favor is that two receptor dimers have to
interact to get a signal transduction mechanism to
work.   Our approach to this problem is to purify

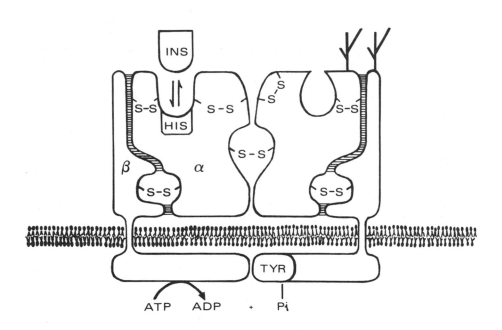

FIG. 1. Structural Features of the Insulin Receptor
     This cartoon depicts the well-known subunit
structure of the insulin receptor. Note the disulfides
shown in the vicinity of the insulin binding pocket.
These are presumably the "crosslinking" disulfides.
The disulfides in the middle of the receptor are class
1 disulphides, those we reduce to obtain functionally
monomeric receptor. The cytoplasmic kinase domain
shows phosphorylation of the opposite half that binds
insulin.   This is for convenience sake and is not
meant to imply any mechanism of autophosphorylation.

receptors, reduce the receptor _via_ the class 1 disulphides, which are readily reducible under mild
conditions, and then analyze the functional properties
of the resulting receptor monomers with regard to
insulin binding and kinase activation.

Now, as you have heard earlier from Dr. Rutter,
there is another class of disulphides which has been
postulated to be involved in insulin binding, that he
has called crosslinking disulphides. I would like to
show you some of our data that tends to suggest that
these disulphides are, in fact, in the binding domain,
and how we can get around the possible confounding
effects when we use dithiothreitol to reduce class I
disulphides. We don't, indeed, reduce the disulphides
in the binding domain.

In the experiment shown here, we have crosslinked
[125]I-insulin to purified human placental insulin
receptor and treated the complex with thermolysin for
the times indicated and it's about a 50-fold molar
excess of thermolysin to receptor. So in 60 to 120
minutes, we see the formation of a rather stable
fragment of about 50,000 molecular weight covalently
linked to insulin. When we treat this fragment with
dithiothreitol, we can see a classic shift in mobility
in SDS-PAGE (see reference 2, FIG. 5, for example).
The dithiothreitol concentrations are added in the
electrophoresis buffer, and as we add increasing
amounts of dithiothreitol, we get first a slight downward shift and then an upward shift in mobility and an
apparent increase in size which is diagnostic for
multiple internal disulphide bonds such as seen in
albumin. A similar sort of phenomenon can be seen in
the intact insulin receptor. So, we think this data
indicates that insulin can be crosslinked to the
vicinity of this so called disulphide crosslinking
domain, and in our subsequent protocols to reduce
receptors into functional halves, we have to take
great care that we don't (in fact) destroy those
particular disulphides which seemed to be directly
involved in the structure of the binding domain. One
trick of the protocol is to use an alkaline pH and low
concentrations of dithiothreitol, and this works with
receptors in membrane as well, and the trick here is
that alkaline pH and low concentrations of DTT favor
not only reduction of disulphides but also reoxidation
of intramolecular disulphides such as one would expect
to see in the so called cross-linking domain of the
receptor. To get rid of the DTT when we are using
membranes, we simply centrifuge. If we are using
purified soluble receptor, we put it over a desalting
column. These procedures eliminate the residual DTT,

and then we do our various assays of insulin binding and autophosphorylation. It is very important that, before we run SDS-PAGE, we add N-ethylmaleimide to freeze any further redox reactions which can take place in SDS, as Jeff Pessin has shown. Then we typically run SDS-PAGE or do Scatchard analyses or what have you.

This experiment is just to show you that our reduction protocol does not, in fact, when applied to intact receptor, lead to a disruption of the intra-molecular disulphides in the binding region (FIG 4, reference 2). We have either reduced receptor as in lanes two or four. In lanes one and two this is a membrane preparation. In lanes three and four this is a purified receptor preparation in detergent. Then we reduced it or not, added ^{125}I-insulin and crosslinked and ran gels in the presence of N-ethylmaleimide. What you can see is that in detergent, when we do this reduction in detergent, we see a shift in apparent mobility diagnostic for reducing the disulphide bonds in the so called crosslinking region. However, when we do it in membranes we don't see any apparent shift in molecular weight and we take this data to mean that our reducing protocols are in fact not terribly damaging to the binding domain of the receptor. We have further evidence for that as you will see in subsequent slides.

So in the next experiment we have retreated mem-branes with dithiothreitol at alkaline pH, briefly centrifuged them, and then done a Scatchard analysis of tracer insulin binding. And in the top of the Figure, the binding is done to the membranes (FIG. 6, reference 2). Whether we treat with reducing agent or not, we see a typical curvilinear Scatchard plot indicating no apparent change in insuln binding para-meters due to this reduction protocol. However, if we take that preparation, add detergent, immobilize on wheat germ and then get the receptor off the wheat germ with N-acetyl glucosamine and then do a binding assay in detergent, we see with the unreduced receptors, the typical type of insulin binding plot, cuvilinear; but with the reduced receptor we see a markedly decreased affinity for ligand and an apparent increase in the stoichiometry of the binding from one apparently high affinity binding site, and one very low affinity binding site to two low affinity binding sites (FIG. 6, reference 2). Now our data are not totally definitive on this matter, but it looks like the stoichiometry of insulin binding is one high affinity binding insulin site per intact receptor and also one per monomeric receptor. Jeff Pessin will also present data which reached the same conclusion.

So, we think that a dimeric receptor structure, two functional monomers, is involved in high affinity binding. What about kinase activation? Well, also just to show that in fact the receptor that we are talking about in detergent is really a monomer and not a dimer, we run it out in sucrose gradient (FIG. 3., reference 1). The bottom of the gradient are low fraction numbers, and the top of the gradient, high numbers. Here is the position of the intact receptor. Here is the position of the receptor monomer, the alpha-beta half, and clearly after reducing the receptor in the membrane, we convert essentially all receptor into this monomeric species. Interestingly enough, something that we have commented on in the lab, in light of Cecil Yip's talk, we always see some high-molecular weight complex at the bottom of the gradient and we don't know what that complex might be. Anyway, to the kinase situation. So, here we have reduced the receptor, run it out in sucrose gradients, added insulin or not, and add gamma-^{32}P-ATP to see what happens (FIG. 5, reference 1). This is the monomeric fraction, the alpha-beta half. In the first series of such experiments that we ran, we were puzzled by the fact that we seemed to see a slight effect of insulin on these receptor monomers. This is the alpha-beta 210 K species, and we see a small degree of apparent reoxidation of receptor monomer to receptor dimer. When one quantitates those values in terms of the insulin effect; here is no insulin, here is insulin receptor in the dimeric form, here is no insulin, here is insulin receptor in the monomeric form and obviously this is a marked stimulation typical of what one sees in an intact receptor. This is a rather marginal insulin effect observed for the half receptor, and we didn't know exactly how to explain this data. About this time, Ray Erikson published sucrose density gradients of the src protein, suggesting that if you didn't include a reasonable concentration of sodium chloride, that you would get aggregation of src. So we reran the same experiments in the presence of sodium chloride (FIGS. 6 and 7, reference 1). This should be the alpha-two beta-two species, the intact receptor, the functionally dimeric form. Here is the half receptor, functionally monomeric form. This is the presence and absence of insulin, and in the presence of gamma-^{32}P-ATP, and you can see a very substantial insulin effect on the intact receptor and essentially no effect on the monomeric receptor. This is quantitated in the same experiment where the bands have been cut out and counted (FIG. 7, 1), and again, you see about a five-fold effect of insulin in the intact receptor on autophosphorylation activity, and no insulin effect for the monomeric receptor.

We did this experiment in a different way. That is, we took receptor and reduced it or not. These are the reduced lanes, A and B and E and F, intact lanes G and H and C and D (FIG. 2. reference 4). The receptor was reduced in the membrane, solubilized in detergent, partially purified on immobilized wheat germ, eluted from the wheat germ, and then in the case of this panel on the left, the receptor was added back to the wheat germ so that the receptor is now immobilized and not free in solution. In the panel on the right, the receptor is still free in solution. Then one adds gamma-^{32}-ATP and insulin, and when the functionally monomeric receptor is bound to wheat germ, there is absolutely no insulin response, whereas the dimeric insulin receptor responds quite nicely. In solution, you see a slightly different effect. Apparently, an insulin response on the monomeric form can occur with some reoxidation as we saw before and, of course, the intact receptor responds to insulin quite nicely. So, if you keep the receptor monomers apart by either salt or by immobilization, they are totally unresponsive to insulin. If they can come together in any way, they are responsive to insulin. And we think this means that, with regard to the model I showed you, insulin binds to presumably only one of two possible sites making the other site one of very low affinity for ligand. The binding causes some conformational changes in the extracellular-domain of the receptor such that the interaction of the two halves probably causes an interaction of these two intracellular halves. I would like to believe that there is some kind of transphosphorylation although we don't have any data for that at this point. In any case, it amounts to an allosterically regulated enzymatic system where insulin is the allosteric regulator that causes an increase in the autophosphorylation activity at the cytoplasmic side of the membrane as the initial event in transmembrane signalling.

The fact that our receptors will readily reoxidize if we don't keep them apart, and readily rerespond to insulin, supports the notion that the chemical modification is not drastic with regard to altering the structure of the receptor. However, as a sort of analogous situation, one can consider the EGF receptor. Here the insulin receptor is a functional dimer covalently linked together. We analyzed it by chemical reduction, but the EGF receptor as you've heard from Dr. Rutter is very similar, in the same family as the insulin receptor, and has this same so-called crosslinking domain but it is not covalently linked by disulphide bonds. So we sought to ask the same kind of questions about the EGF receptor as the insulin receptor. If you look (FIG. 1, reference 3), and this is detergent solubilized EGF receptor from A431 cells run through a sucrose gradient (dimer near the bottom of the gradient, monomer near the top) and assayed by measuring tracer binding, you see two peaks. This corresponds to the monomeric EGF receptor molecular weight of 170,000, this is the dimeric form of 340,000, approximately the same size as the insulin receptor in sucrose, and if you Western-blot for EGF receptors across this gradient, you see a very good signal corresponding to the monomer but you see virtually nothing where you have a substantial amount of tracer binding to the dimer. One possible explanation for this is that the dimer binds with higher affinity just as we suggested was the case for the insulin receptor. So we isolated EGF receptor forms and did Scatchard analysis of EGF binding to the dimer and to the monomer (FIG. 2, reference 3), and sure enough, you see a substantially higher affinity of the dimer for EGF as compared to the monomer. The number of binding sites are irrelevant in this particular case since we didn't normalize for equivalent numbers of binding sites for monomer and dimer.

Well, what is the effect of EGF in this system? What EGF does, and these are EGF receptors purified from A431 cells not treated with EGF, this is treated with EGF, and then run on sucrose gradients (FIG. 5, reference 3). What EGF does is convert monomers to dimers. So the EGF receptor system is very analagous in some ways and a little different in other ways to the insulin/IGF-1 receptor systems. We have done kinase measurements on monomers and dimers. The dimers are intrinsically activated for the EGF receptor. They don't respond, or minimally respond, to EGF., Rather the monomers respond to EGF and the way the monomers respond is by converting to dimers, the dimers being constitutively active in terms of autophosphorylation (3).

Table 1 is a summary of our data on the functional properties of the insulin (IR) and epidermal growth factor receptors (EGFR). In both cases, the EGF and insulin receptors, the monomer has low affinity for a ligand, the dimer has a high affinity. The kinase activity, the autophosphorylation activity of the monomer is low in the absence of ligand. In the case of the EGF dimer, it is high and in the case of the

TABLE 1. Functional properties of receptor/kinases

| | IR | | EGFR | |
	monomer	dimer	monomer	dimer
High affinity ligand binding	no	yes	no	yes
High Intrinsic autophos. capacity	no	no	no	yes
Ligand-stimulated autophos. response.	no	yes	yes	no
Enhanced exogenous kinase activity after autophos.	yes	yes	?	?

insulin receptor only the dimer responds to insulin. The insulin receptor monomer, however, can form a non-covalently associated dimer that will then be able to respond to insulin. This is somewhat similar to the EGF receptor where the monomeric form responds to ligand by dimerization. This mechanism, we would postulate, is also operating *in vivo* for the EGF receptor, and there are much indirect data to support this postulate from numerous labs. If the insulin receptor is autophosphorylated in the presence of ligand, and then reduced, the resultant monomer is still fully active towards exogenous substrates (last row of the table). It appears that the kinase domain of the insulin receptor, once phosphorylated, is independent of the rest of the receptor molecule, and is highly activated towards reporter substrates. There is not yet available, unequivocal data on this point for the EGF receptor. The effects of ligand on the various EGF and insulin receptor forms are also shown schematically in figure 2.

In summary, I hope I have convinced you that for this particular class of receptors, the initial event in the ligand-dependent biological activity is the transmembrane activation of autophosphorylation which occurs by the interaction of two receptor halves. We have some data on this point for the IGF I receptor that we don't show. It seems to parallel the insulin receptor. There is plenty of data in the literature to suggest that the nerve growth factor receptor seems

to be dimeric, homo-dimeric, in order to mediate biological activity (5). A totally different system, the
interleukin-2 receptors seems to need heterologous
dimerization as a requirement for high affinity
binding and ligand activation (6). So as in certain
personal relationships, the interaction of two
partners is critically important for subsequent
biological activity.

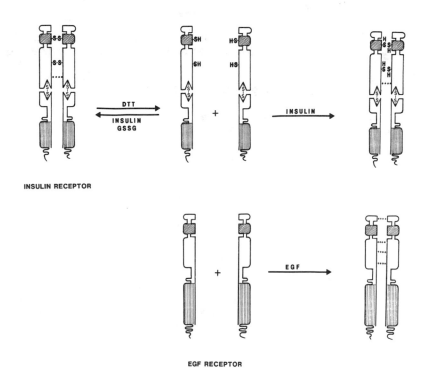

Figure 2. The effect of ligand on receptor form. GSSG
stands for oxidized glutathione.

REFERENCES

1. Boni-Schnetzler, M., Rubin, J.B. and Pilch, P.F. (1986), J. Biol. Chem., 261:15281-15287.

2. Boni-Schnetzler, M., Scott, W., Waugh, S.M., Dibella, E. and Pilch, P.F. (1987), J. Biol. Chem., 262:8395-8401.

3. Boni-Schnetzler, M. and Pilch, P.F. (1987), Proc. Nat. Acad. Sci. U.S.A., 84:7832-7836.

4. Boni-Schnetzler, M., Kaligian, A., DelVecchio, R. and Pilch, P.F. (1987), submitted for publication.

5. Buxser, S. Puma, P. and Johnson, G.L. (1985), J. Biol. Chem., 260:9117-1926.

6. Wang, H.-M., and Smith, K.A. (1987), J. Exp. Med., 166:1055-1069.

Insulin Action and Diabetes,
edited by H. Joseph Goren et al.
Raven Press, New York © 1988.

Isolation of Functional $\alpha\beta$ Heterodimers From The Purified $\alpha_2\beta_2$ Heterotetrameric Human Placental Insulin Receptor Complex

Jeffrey E. Pessin, Laurel J. Sweet[*] and Brian D. Morrison

The Department of Physiology & Biophysics,
The University of Iowa, Iowa City, IA 52242.
[*]Department of Cellular and Developmental Biology,
Harvard University, 16 Divinity Ave., Cambridge, MA 02138.

To address the role of subunit communication in the insulin-dependent transmembrane regulation of insulin receptor function, we have isolated a functional $\alpha\beta$ heterodimeric insulin receptor complex from the purified human placental $\alpha_2\beta_2$ heterotetrameric disulfide-linked state. This has been accomplished by a simultaneous treatment of the purified $\alpha_2\beta_2$ heterotetrameric insulin receptor complex with a combination of alkaline pH (8.50-8.75) and 2.0 mM DTT similar to the method previously described by Boni-Schnetzler et al. (1). The dissociated $\alpha\beta$ heterodimers can then be readily separated from any remaining DTT-treated but nondissociated $\alpha_2\beta_2$ heterotetrameric complexes by rapid Sephadex G-50 and Bio-Gel A-1.5m gel filtration chromatography at 4^0C in a pH 7.6 buffer. The specific isolation of these species was confirmed by nonreducing and reducing SDS-polyacrylamide gel electrophoresis for both ^{125}I-insulin affinity labeled and ^{32}P-autophosphorylated insulin receptor complexes (6).

Competition of insulin binding to the isolated $\alpha_2\beta_2$ heterotetrameric insulin receptor complex produced an apparent curvilinear Scatchard plot with an extremely sharp break compared to that typically observed for intact cells, membrane or partially purified insulin receptor preparations (Fig. 1). Insulin binding was generally found to be linear over the concentration range from 0.1 to 10 nM, similar to other studies (3,4). However, at insulin concentrations above 10 nM, a sharp break in the insulin binding curve was readily apparent. The high and low affinity dissociation constants determined by a two-site binding model were 0.14 ± 0.03 and 37 ± 7, respectively. Saturation of insulin binding in these experiments occurred at approximately 3 nmol of insulin bound/mg of insulin receptor protein, corresponding to 1 mol insulin bound/mol $\alpha_2\beta_2$ heterotetrameric complex. In contrast, Scatchard analysis of insulin binding to the $\alpha\beta$ heterodimeric complex generated a nearly linear plot over the entire insulin concentration range examined, with saturation of insulin binding occurring at approximately 6 nmol/mg, corresponding to 1 mol insulin bound/mol of $\alpha\beta$ heterodimeric complex. These data suggest that the $\alpha_2\beta_2$ heterotetrameric insulin receptor complex exhibits half-site binding reactivity but once dissociated into an $\alpha\beta$ heterodimeric state each α subunit is functionally equivalent with respect to insulin binding. Further, these results are consistent with the high affinity curvilinear binding observed in the $\alpha_2\beta_2$ heterotetrameric insulin receptor complex being a function of intramolecular subunit interactions (2).

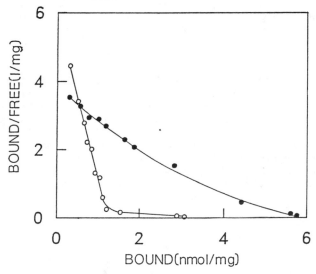

Fig. 1. Scatchard analyses of insulin binding to the isolated $\alpha_2\beta_2$ heterotetrameric (o) and $\alpha\beta$ heterodimeric (•) insulin receptor complexes. Quantitation of the amount of the insulin receptor complexes isolated from the Bio-Gel A-1.5m columns was based upon the known amount of starting material and recovery of ^{32}P-autophosphorylated insulin receptors which were run in parallel.

We next examined the insulin-dependent β subunit autophosphorylation of the isolated $\alpha_2\beta_2$ heterotetrameric and $\alpha\beta$ heterodimeric complexes (Fig. 2A). Autophosphorylation of the $\alpha_2\beta_2$ heterotetrameric complex in the presence of insulin typically resulted in a 2 to 3-fold increase in the initial rate of insulin receptor self-phosphorylation (Fig. 2A, lanes 1 and 2). Reducing SDS-polyacrylamide gel electrophoresis demonstrated that the insulin receptor autophosphorylation occurred exclusively on the β subunit (Fig. 2A, lanes 3 and 4). However, autophosphorylation of the $\alpha\beta$ heterodimeric insulin receptors in the presence of insulin generated the appeearence of a ^{32}P-labeled M_r = 400,000 $\alpha_2\beta_2$ heterotetrameric complex which was barely detectable in the absence of insulin. (Fig. 2B, lanes 1 and 2). Reducing SDS-polyacrylamide gel electrophoresis demonstrated that the insulin-dependent reassociated form was also autophosphorylated on the M_r = 95,000 β subunit (Fig. 2B, lanes 3 and 4). These results are consistent with previous studies suggesting that the $\alpha_2\beta_2$ heterotetrameric complex is the most active insulin-dependent protein kinase species (1,5). Further, these results document that the insulin-dependent transmembrane activation of the insulin receptor kinase also requires intramolecular subunit interaction within the native $\alpha_2\beta_2$ heterotetrameric disulfide-linked complex.

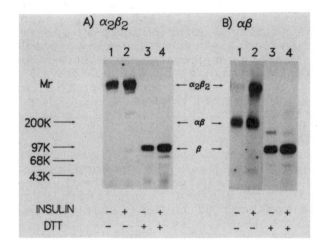

Fig. 2. Insulin-dependent autophosphorylation of the $\alpha_2\beta_2$ heterotetrameric (A) and $\alpha\beta$ heterodimeric (B) insulin receptor complexes. Autophosphorylation was carried out for 5 min in the absence (lanes 1 and 3) or presence (lanes 2 and 4) of 200 nM insulin. The gels were run in the absence (lanes 1 and 2) or presence (lanes 3 and 4) of 100 mM DTT.

REFERENCES

1. Boni-Schnetzler, M., Rubin, J.B. and Pilch, P.F. (1986) J. Biol. Chem. 261, 15281-15287
2. Boni-Schnetzler, M., Scott, W., Waugh, S.M., Dibella, E. and Pilch, P.F. (1987) J. Biol. Chem. 262, 8395-8401
3. Fujita-Yamaguchi, Y. (1984) J. Biol. Chem. 259 1206-1211
4. Kohanski, R.A. and Lane, M.D. (1983) J. Biol. Chem. 258, 7460-7468
5. Shia, M.A., Rubin, J.B. and Pilch, P.F. (1983) J. Biol. Chem. 258, 14450-14455
6. Sweet, L.J., Morrison, B.D. and Pessin, J.E. (1987) J. Biol. Chem. 262, 6939-6942

DISCUSSION (to papers by P. Pilch and J. Pessin)

Dr. Jarett, The University of Pennsylvania. These are both very eloquent presentations. My question is really addressed I guess to both of you, Paul particularly. You demonstrated that with the low DDT that there was a drop in the Scatchard plot, and Jeff, I think yours went up and linearised. Steve Jacobs had reported previously with placenta membranes that low DDT treatment had linearised it but dropped it, and we had prior to that time had reported with fat membranes and liver membrane that when we treated it with DDT that we linearized with very low concentrations. We did linearize the fat cell and it increased and went up, whereas no change occurred what-so-ever with liver membrane binding. At the same time we saw morphologically that the aggregates that seemed to be held together in fat membranes by disulphides of some type were now almost all single receptors; that is based on binding with ferritin-insulin. How do you, particularly Paul, correlate your placental versus the adipocyte model?

Well, there are a couple of things. First, in most of the previous studies , the protocols, unlike, the ones that Jeff and I just described, were done at physiological pH where I think Jeff would agree we both see a somewhat of the unfolding of the binding domain of the insulin receptor so that right away could confound the results. Secondly, there is tissue variability and Jeff can speak to this. All I can say is the major concerns we had were to devise a protocol that had the minimum amount of structural perturbation while leading to a dissociation of dimers to monomers, and I think we succeeded at that. Where there are a lot of previous studies and I don't think they have addressed every issue that we have and so depending on the tissue, you'll get different results and Jeff has some data on it. (P. Pilch)

We have some data that addresses that actually. We have done very similar studies on adipocyte membranes and we get exactly what you see. We see an increase in high affinity binding and it becomes very very steep, but as we purify the adipocyte receptor, we don't see that phenomenon. It looks just like the placenta. So placenta membranes and purified human insulin receptors behave in this phenomenon. Purified adipocyte receptor also behaves in this manner, but adipocyte membrane bound receptors do not, and we are currently studying that. We don't know what it is,

but it is something to do with the membrane.   It is
something in the membrane environment which alters the
properties of the receptor binding and kinase
activity. (J. Pessin)

Possibly the clusters that you (Dr. Jarett) report
and which we would expect to have higher affinity
binding. (P. Pilch)

L. Jarett, Philadelphia. That's right. Which do
disappear because we tried to isolate many times those
clusters by solubilizing the adipocyte membrane, and
we kept putting them through columns and everything
else. We have never been able to find the aggregates
that we see morphologically.

R. Kahn, Boston. I have a short question for Paul. On
the very last summary table you showed there was the
column related to exogenous kinase activity, and it
was going quickly, but I thought it said that both the
monomer and the dimer had high exogenous kinase
activity.

I think the function that was measured was exogenous kinase activity of autophosphorylated receptor.
The way that that was done was that the receptor dimer
was fully autophosphorylated and then reduced or not
so to see whether the reduction protocol had any
affect, per se, on this activated kinase activity and
it did not. The dimer and the monomer were equally
active. If anything, the monomer after autophosphorylation was a little more active. I didn't show that
data. (P. Pilch)

R. Kahn, Boston. So, then the conclusion to put that
in context with the autophosphorylation is that you
would feel that the monomer is not able to undergo a
full activation of autophosphorylation. If it could
be autophosphorylated, it would be fully active as a
kinase on exogenous substrate.

Exactly. (P. Pilch)

M. Hollenberg, Calgary. Just a quick question. Way up
front, Paul, you talked about the use of NEM and then
kind of didn't mention it for the rest of your talk.
I am wondering if all of the experiments that you did
were quenched with NEM? All the gels were quenched
with NEM.

That is correct. (P. Pilch)

M. Hollenberg, Calgary. But not the kinase?

No, the NEM will inhibit the kinase activity (P. Pilch)

M. Hollenberg, Calgary. Right.

And we did verify, for example doing kinase assays with soluble receptor, that we could get rid of about 99% of the DTT to such a degree that we couldn't measure any effect of it on binding or anything or on insulin itself. (P. Pilch)

M. Hollenberg, Calgary. So in summary, all of the functional assays, phosphorylation or binding, were done without NEM treatment, gel analyses with NEM treatment.

Correct. (P. Pilch)

J. Avruch, Boston. Question for Paul. In the EGF data that you presented you said that the dimeric EGF receptor will autophosphorylate and I guess will be a kinase and it doesn't require EGF in order to do so.

That is correct. The EGF stimulation that we see on the dimeric form varies from nil up to two fold. (P. Pilch)

J. Avruch, Boston. How does the activity compare to a comparable number of receptors to which EGF is added?

Right. We did exactly that experiment. We normalized it. It's as high or higher. If you take one mole of monomers and add EGF to it and one mole of dimers, the monomers will presumably dimerize to half a mole and have half or less the activity of a mole of already formed dimers (P. Pilch).

J. Avruch, Boston. Have you been able to add insulin to a low enough concentration of EGF receptors so that EGF will bind but dimerization cannot occur?

I'm sorry. Add insulin to EGF receptors? (P. Pilch)

J. Avruch, Boston. Is the receptor present at a low enough concentration that dimerization is impaired and then add EGF and examine the kinase?

Yes. We have done a few of those, and I think Yosi

Yarden and Yosi Schlessinger just published on this. If you do that, you see that the receptor autophosphorylation reaction seems to be EGF receptor-concentration dependent as you would expect for the dimer complex to form. (P. Pilch)

Thank You. (P. Pilch)

Insulin Action and Diabetes,
edited by H. Joseph Goren et al.
Raven Press, New York © 1988.

ELECTRICAL EVENTS IN TRANSDUCTION OF INSULIN ACTION

AND INSULIN ACTION ON ELECTRICAL EVENTS

Kenneth Zierler

Department of Medicine, The Johns Hopkins University
School of Medicine, 718 Traylor Building, 720 Rutland
Avenue, Baltimore, MD 21205

I am going to consider,first, some mechanisms of
insulin action, involving ion currents and electrical
potential in transduction of insulin signals,
and,second, our recent work on effects of insulin on
some ion channels newly recognized in skeletal
muscle.

In nature, forces are dichotomized as strong or
weak. Electrical potential gradients are classified
among the strong forces. There is an electrical
potential difference across surface membranes of all
true cells in animals, whether or not the cells are
excitable, like nerve and muscle. Among these
various types of cells, the difference in electrical
potential between cytosol and extracellular fluid
covers a narrow range from about -40 to -90 mV, the
inside being negative with respect to the outside.
This electrical potential difference is across the
cell membrane, some 60 to 90 A. The electrical
potential gradient, or the electrical field strength,
is therefore of the order of 100,000 V/cm. This is
an enormous force, more than 100 times the force we
use in our ordinary laboratory electrophoresis. We
may wonder why cells such as hepatocytes and
adipocytes go to all that trouble and expense, but
that is another story.

There are phenomena in cells well-known to be
sensitive to small changes in transmembrane
electrical potential difference. For example, the
rate at which Na^+ ions pass through the tetrodotoxin-
(TTX)-sensitive Na^+ channel doubles for only about 2
mV depolarization.

INSULIN HYPERPOLARIZES SKELETAL AND CARDIAC MUSCLE
AND ADOPOCYTES

In the 1950's I found that insulin hyperpolarized rat skeletal muscle (13). The observation has been confirmed in a number of laboratories in rat , mouse, and frog muscle (3,4,7,8,12). Insulin-induced hyperpolarization, IIH, is reported in adipose tissue and adipocytes (1,2,9), and in canine and chick heart (5,6). In rat caudofemoralis muscle, maximum IIH is by 8-10 mV. Half-maximum IIH occurs at an insulin concentration of 30-100 μU/ml, about 0.2-0.7 *nM*.

HYPERPOLARIZATION IS PROBABLY A LINK IN THE INSULIN
TRANSDUCTION CHAIN LEADING TO GLUCOSE UPTAKE

After a number of years it finally dawned on me that the hyperpolarization induced by insulin might be one step in the transduction chain between the initial association of insulin with its receptor and the final stimulation of specific D-glucose transport. If hyperpolarization is a transduction step, then three conditions must be met:

1)Insulin must hyperpolarize in less time than is required to stimulate glucose uptake. This seems to be the case. Insulin hyperpolarizes in less than 1 sec (18). I have seen it in less than 500 msec. Noone has reported insulin-stimulated glucose uptake in less than about 50 sec, 100 times the interval required to hyperpolarize. The caution is that one can get much better time resolution with measurements of membrane potential than with measurements of glucose transport.

2)One should be able to carry out the same kind of experiment as one does with a chain of chemical events. If one thinks that B may be an intermediate between A and C, A-->B-->C, then one ought to be able to dispense with A, simply administer B, and examine whether or not C occurs. With a triple sucrose-gap apparatus, Ellen Rogus and I found that, without any insulin, with only 2 or 3 mV of electrically-produced hyperpolarization (which is only about 1/5 to 1/3 of that produced by insulin, but which was all we could achieve with the apparatus), D-glucose uptake increased by 40% (16). This was stereospecific; L-glucose uptake was not affected.

3)Finally, if hyperpolarization is a transduction step leading to increased glucose transport, then we must find a way to intervene at a step preceding hyperpolarization, so that insulin does not

hyperpolarize, and observe whether insulin then fails
to stimulate glucose uptake. We exclude the trivial
case in which insulin is not able to combine with its
receptor.   Ellen Rogus , Bobbi Scherer,Fong-Sen Wu
and I found that insulin depolarizes to a lesser
extent as muscles are bathed in increasing potassiun
concentration, and that, correlated with this, there
was decreased responsiveness with respect to glucose
uptake (19).
     There is, then, a body of evidence suggesting,
some of it strongly, that hyperpolarization is a step
in   the   transduction   chain.   Granting   that
hyperpolarization is a transduction step, we can
exploit that opportunity to reveal neighboring steps,
and so hope to work our way, step-by-step, back to
the   receptor   and   down   to   stimulated   glucose
transport.   Let's begin with the step immediately
leading to hyperpolarization.

THE IMMEDIATE MECHANISM FOR INSULIN-INDUCED HYPERPOLARIZATION OF RAT SKELETAL MUSCLE

     What is the immediate mechanism by which insulin
hyperpolarizes? The possibilities fall into two
categories. The membrane potential can be considered
the weighted sum of two components in parallel: an
electrogenic pump, V_P, and a diffusive component, V_D:

$$V_m = T_P V_P + T_D V_D .$$

The T's are partial conductances, the relative
contribution of the given potential component to
total conductance through the membrane. The
electrogenic pump pumps out more Na^+ than it pumps in
K^+. It is inhibited by ouabain. The diffusive
component is given by the classical Goldman-Hodgkin-
Katz equation:

$$V_D = -(RT/F) \ln \frac{P_K [K^+]_i + P_{Na} [Na^+]_i + P_{Cl} [Cl^-]_o}{P_K [K^+]_o + P_{Na} [Na^+]_o + P_{Cl} [Cl^-]_i},$$

a   constant,   consisting   of   the   gas   constant,
temperature, and the Faraday constant, is multiplied
by the logarithm of a ratio representing the weighted
sum of ion activities tending to cause outward
electrical current and the weighted sum of ions
tending to cause inward current. The weighting
factors, the P's, are permeability coefficients for
the indicated ion through the cell membrane under
study. The size of the diffusive component can be

changed by altering ion concentrations or by altering permeabilities.

Let's now consider evidence for and against these possible mechanisms by which insulin hyperpolarizes.

There are reports, based on use of ouabain, mainly by Richard Moore and his colleagues (7) and by Torben Clausen and his colleagues (4), interpreted to mean that insulin hyperpolarizes by stimulating the Na^+-K^+ pump. There are other reports that ouabain has no effect on IIH (6,8). Unequivocal proof that insulin hyperpolarizes by stimulating an electrogenic pump would be that the membrane potential in the presence of insulin became more hyperpolarized than the K^+ equilibrium potential, E_K, but noone has reported such an occurrence when the bathing solution has a normal electrolyte composition. In rat skeletal muscle Ellen Rogus and I (17) found that ouabain, under what we define as appropriate conditions for its use, does not prevent or reduce IIH. Isoproterenol, a β-adrenergic agonist, hyperpolarizes rat skeletal muscle by stimulating the Na^+-K^+ pump. ouabain, 10^{-6} M, reduces isoproterenol-induced hyperpolarization by 50%; $10^{-5} M$ blocks it entirely within 5-10 minutes. But even $10^{-4} M$ ouabain has no effect on IIH during that time period. We conclude that IIH is not caused by stimulation of an electrogenic pump.

In skeletal muscle it is generally held that there is no Cl^- pump; Cl^- is distributed only passively in accordance with its electrochemical potential gradient. Therefore, the terms in $[Cl^-]$ can be dropped from the equation for V_D, so that we now have:

$$V_D = -(RT/F)\ln\frac{[K^+]_i + (P_{Na}/P_K)[Na^+]_i}{[K^+]_o + (P_{Na}/P_K)[Na^+]_o}.$$

The ratio P_{Na}/P_K is about 0.01-0.02 in rat skeletal muscle. The membrane potential is less polarized than E_K. If P_{Na} were zero, the membrane potential would be E_K. In rat skeletal muscle at rest the membrane potential is not affected by ouabain, up to $10^{-4} M$ for 10 min. Therefore, in this muscle $V_m = V_D$ at rest.

If insulin hyperpolarizes by increasing the potential due to the diffusive component, it must do so by increasing the ratio of $[K^+]_i/[K^+]_o$ or by decreasing the ratio of Na^+/K^+ permeability. We have known for 50 years that insulin reduces K^+ concentration in blood serum and later we learned that insulin redistributes K from extracellular to intracellular space. But this is not the cause of IIH. Studies of the time course of IIH and of the shift in K showed that hyperpolarization preceded the shift in K (14), that the shift in K could not account quantitatively for the hyperpolarization and that it was the other way around: the insulin-induced redistribution of K is accounted for quantitatively and temporally by the observed hyperpolarization.

This leaves only the possibility that insulin hyperpolarizes by decreasing the ratio P_{Na}/P_K, which has the effect of driving the membrane potential away from the Na^+ equilibrium potential toward the K^+ equilibrium potential. When P_{Na} is zero, the membrane potential equals E_K. The ratio P_{Na}/P_K can decrease either because P_{Na} decreases or P_K increases, or by any combination of changes in both P_{Na} and P_K that leads to a decreases ratio. Lantz, Elsas and DeHaan (6) interpreted their experiments on cultured embryonic chick cardiocytes to mean that insulin hyperpolarized those cells by increasing K^+ conductance or P_K.

However, our own data, on ^{42}K flux from rat skeletal muscle showed that insulin decreases P_K. That being so, the only way in which insulin could hyperpolarize muscle under the scheme we have been considering is to decrease P_{Na} even more, so that the ratio P_{Na}/P_K becomes smaller. If this is the explanation, then V_m should, as it does, approach but not exceed E_K.

The modified Goldman-Hodgkin-Katz equation is rearranged to solve explicitly for P_{Na}/P_K:

$$P_{Na}/P_K = ([K^+]_i e^x - [K^+]_o)/([Na^+]_o - [Na^+]_i e^x),$$

where $x = FV_D/RT$. Because $[Na^+]_i$ is small compared to $[Na^+]_o$ and $x<0$, under normal conditions the term $[Na^+]_i e^x$ is negligible compared to $[Na^+]_o$, and the ratio is given approximately by

$$P_{Na}/P_K \approx ([K^+]_i e^x - [K^+]_o)/[Na^+]_o.$$

All components on the right-hand side are measurable experimentally. In normal Krebs-Ringer-HCO_3 solution, average V_m in rat caudofemoralis muscle is $-78mV$ and P_{Na}/P_K is about 0.02; P_K is 50 times P_{Na}. Half-maximum hyperpolarization by insulin reduces P_{Na}/P_K in half; P_K is 100 times P_{Na}. At maximum response to insulin, P_{Na}/P_K is reduced to 0.0024; P_K is 400 times P_{Na}.

Recently, Fong-Sen Wu and I (11) have carried out a series of experiments which could settle the question of the immediate mechanism of IIH, and which, in conjunction with data from our earlier experiments, leads to calculations of the effect of insulin on P_K and, separately, on P_{Na}. Substitute some large poorly permeant cation for Na^+ in the bathing solution. Call this ion B^+. P_B is substantially less than P_{Na}. The Goldman-Hodgkin Katz equation is then modified to

$$V_D = -(RT/F)\ln\frac{P_K[K^+]_i + P_B[B^+]_i + P_{Cl}[Cl^-]_o}{P_K[K^+]_o + P_B[B^+]_o + P_{Cl}[Cl^-]_i}.$$

If $P_B = 0$ and if Cl^- is distributed purely passively, so that E_{Cl} assumes whatever value V_D has, then V_D is just E_K. In this case, if the hypothesis is correct, then insulin will not change the membrane potential because any effect of P_K cancels out of the numerator and denominator of the logarithmic term. But if P_B is not zero and if insulin has no effect on P_B, the hypothesis predicts that insulin will depolarize, instead of hyperpolarizing, because it will decrease P_K. The beauty of the experiment is that it distinguishes clearly between our hypothesis that insulin decreases the ratio P_{Na}/P_K by decreasing both P's, but decreases P_{Na} to a relatively greater extent, and the two other hypotheses, that insulin increases P_K or that insulin stimulates the Na^+-K^+ pump. If insulin hyperpolarizes by either of these latter two mechanisms, it should still do so in the absence of extracellular Na, provided that, for the hypothesis that P_K increases, P_B is not zero.

Some of the results appear in Table 1. Either TRIS or *N*-methylglucamine was substituted for Na in the bathing solution. All other ions normally in Krebs-Ringer solution, except HCO_3, were present. Data in Table 1 are from TRIS experiments, but results were similar with *N*-methylglucamine. The protocol was as follows: First, there was a period during which the muscles were bathed only in Na^+-free TRIS. Some 10-20 measurements of V_m were made over a period of about 10 min. Then, in a second period, either nothing was added (a time control) or additions were made as shown in the left-hand column, and measurements of V_m were repeated. In both cases the membrane potential of rat caudofemoralis muscle became more negative than in normal Na solutions, showing that P_B for both these large cations is smaller than P_{Na}.

TABLE 1. *Effect of Na⁺-free solution on membrane potential of rat caudofemoralis muscle, and on insulin action on membrane potential.*

Addition 2nd period	Membrane potential, mV		
	1st period	2nd period	Difference
None	-82.3 ± 1.8 (4)	-82.6 ± 2.5	N.S.
Valinomycin	-83.2 ± 0.6 (6)	-89.6 ± 0.4	-6.4 ± 0.56
9ACA	-82.5 ± 0.8 (7)	-81.9 ± 0.7	N.S.
Insulin	-82.8 ± 0.9 (9)	-79.3 ± 0.8	3.5 ± 0.86

Data are means±standard error. Number of muscles is in parenthesis. Difference is 2nd period minus 1st. N.S. is not significant.

However, neither P_B was zero, a fact demonstrated by the observation that V_m was not as polarized as E_K; when valinomycin was added to the Na⁺-free solution, V_m became still more negative. When the Cl⁻ channel blocker 9-anthracenecarboxylic acid (9ACA) was added to the Na⁺-free solution there was no efffect on V_D, validating that we can ignore the Cl⁻ terms. When insulin was added to either Na⁺-free solution the membrane was depolarized, instead of hyperpolarized, compatible with an insulin-induced decrease in P_K.

We can now quantitate the effect of insulin on P_{Na}. If we make the reasonable assumption that insulin had no effect on permeability of either of these substituted large cations, then P_K was decreased by about 40% in the absence of Na⁺. If the same decrease in P_K is produced by insulin in normal Krebs-Ringer solution, then insulin decreased P_{Na} by a factor of 13. Na⁺ permeability is 13 times larger in the absence of insulin than in its presence.

Thus there is strong evidence that the step in the transduction chain immediately preceding hyperpolarization is a reduction in permeability to both Na⁺ and K⁺, with decreased ratio of P_{Na}/P_K due to a major effect on Na⁺ permeability.

INSULIN INCREASES CURRENT THROUGH A NA⁺-CURRENT-DEPENDENT EARLY OUTWARD K⁺ CHANNEL IN RAT MYOBALLS

To get further insight into this process we turned to experiments on primary cultures of embryonic rat skeletal muscle, intending to observe insulin effects on single ion channels. We were soon diverted by an unexpected finding that has no obvious relationship to insulin-induced hyperpolarization, but which is an effect of insulin on an ion channel.

Fong-Sen Wu and I were studying rat myoballs. A myoball is formed when myotubes are treated with colchicine. The long, thin, slightly fusiform muscle fibers are changed into spheres, the diameters of which can be controlled to some extent by the protocol of exposure to colchicine. We aim for about 30 μm diameter. We use patch-clamp electrodes in the whole cell mode. A small pipette, filled with an "intracellular" solution and connected electrically to a suitable circuit, is manipulated to the surface of a myoball. Suction is applied to form a seal between cell and glass of some 10-20 GΩ. With further suction the membrane ruptures, and the contents of pipette and cell intermingle. Because pipette volume is many times greater than cell volume, the composition of the cell interior is also under experimental control. When a voltage is applied between pipette and a reference electrode in the bath, the entire cell membrane is clamped at that voltage, where it stays as long as that voltage is maintained. The current recorded passes through every open channel in the cell; it is self-integrated.

Each frame in Figure 1 displays records from a single cell; current as a function of time. The cell is clamped at a holding potential, V_H, where it is held until a square-wave voltage change is made, e.g. to -40 mV, maintained for,say, 30 or 300 msec.Currents in response to eight such depolarization steps are superimposed in the top frames in Fig 1. Inward currents are downward. The rapid initial outward current is the capacitative current, not due to passage of ions through the membrane. It is followed immediately by a large transient inward current, the tetrodotoxin-, TTX, sensitive Na^+ current, which is off scale in three of the four frames. The Na^+ current is followed usually in adult skeletal muscle by an exponentially-rising, monotonic non-decreasing, outward current which plateaus and persists, shown on the two right-hand frames. This is the major K^+ current, the delayed rectifier. However, in about 75% of the myoballs there is an early transient outward current, shown in the two left-hand frames. This current fuses at onset with the tail of the Na^+ current and then rises rapidly above what will be the plateau of the delayed rectifier and falls quickly to fuse with the rising phase or plateau of the delayed rectifier. This is a

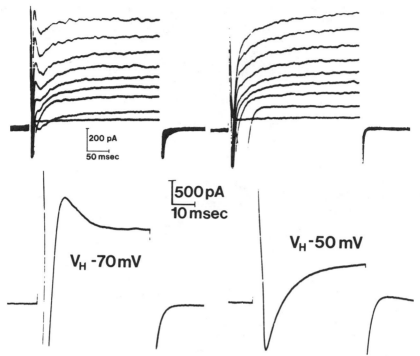

FIG. 1. *Whole cell currents in rat myoballs, showing the early outward transient K⁺ current.*

K⁺ current Fong-Sen Wu and I (10) have recently discovered. This K⁺ current has the most unusual property of undergoing transition from the closed, non-conducting, state to the open, conducting, state in response to passage of current through the TTX-dependent Na⁺ channel. It is a Na⁺-conductance dependent K⁺ current, denoted by $I_K(Na)$.

In Fig 2 are displayed whole cell currents from a single myoball. The two left-hand frames display records in the absence of insulin; the two right-hand frames, in the presence of insulin. The two top frames were recorded under conditions in which $I_K(Na)$ was present in the control; the two bottom frames, under conditions in which $I_K(Na)$ was not present in the control. When there was $I_K(Na)$ in controls it was obviously increased by insulin. When there was no $I_K(Na)$ in the control (as was the case when V_H was too small to activate a sufficiently large number of Na⁺ channels) insulin caused $I_K(Na)$ to appear (20). Insulin had no effect on Na⁺ current. Therefore, insulin, or one of its messengers, increases $I_K(Na)$

by some means other than by increasing current
through the TTX-sensitive Na⁺ channel.

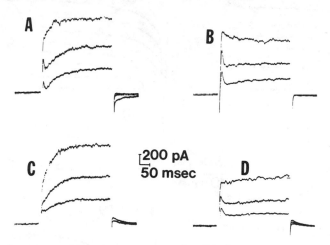

FIG. 2. *Insulin increases* $I_K(Na)$.

What is the function of this $I_K(Na)$? It is the
earliest outward ionic current. It is, therefore,
the current which first opposes the Na⁺ inward
current responsible for the rising phase of the
action potential. Its function may be expected to be
to initiate the repolarization phase of the action
potential, and we have carried out experiments which
seem to support this conjecture.

From this experience we expect that insulin might
accelerate repolarization, and it seems to. Fig 3
displays records from one cell. These are superimposed action potentials of rat myoballs held under
current-clamp. The record in the absence of insulin
is displayed as a dotted line; that in the presence
of insulin by a continuous line. Resting potential
was -59 mV in the control and -63 mV with insulin.
Current was injected (at a time earlier than shown on
these records) and action potentials were generated.
There is a rapid rise to a relatively sharp peak,
followed by a slower fall toward the resting level.
Time required to fall halfway to complete
repolarization is typically only about 2 msec. Two
features are to be noted: The action potential in the
presence of insulin is larger. It is larger because
insulin has hyperpolarized, and so has actvated more
Na⁺ channels. Repolarization is more rapid in the
presence of insulin; the time required for the action
potential to fall to half its peak value is greater
in the control.

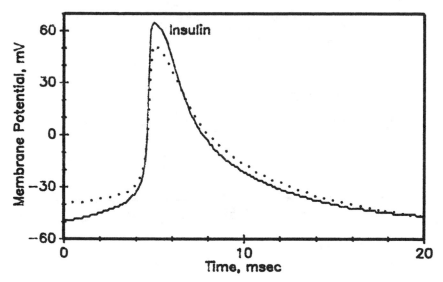

FIG. 3. *Effect of insulin on action potentials.*

ADDENDUM: INSULIN DECREASES A LATE, LONG-LASTING CA^{2+}
CURRENT IN RAT MYOBALLS.

Subsequent to this Symposium, Fong-Sen Wu and I
wanted to observe the effect on the action potential
of eliminating all outward K^+ currents. To this end,
Cs^+ was substituted for K^+ in the pipette. The
skeletal muscle action potential now resembled a
myocardial action potential. There was a long plateau
phase shortly after the peak of the action potential,
lasting for about one second. We demonstrated that
the plateau phase of the myoball action potential in
the absence of K^+ currents is due to a long-lasting
inward Ca^{2+} current. Fig 4 shows the effect of
insulin on this long-lasting Ca^{2+} current, which is
unmasked when outward K^+ currents are eliminated by
substituting Cs^+ for intracellular K^+. On the left
are whole-cell currents under voltage clamp. During a
300 msec depolarizing pulse there is, in the control,
a long-lasting, rather large inward Ca^{2+} current over
the entire period. Insulin, added to the same cell in
nM concentration, reduces this Ca^{2+} current greatly.
On the right, from the same cell, are the
corresponding action potentials under current clamp,
showing the prolonged (1 sec) action potential in the
control. Insulin reduces the duration of this plateau
to nearly one third, more effectively than the

conventional Ca^{2+}-channel blocker, nimodipine, which requires 100 times the insulin concentration to achieve the same effect.

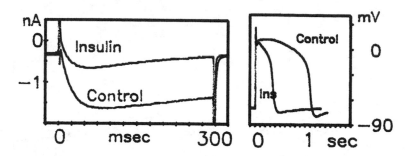

FIG. 4. *Insulin decreases the Ca^{2+} current responsible for the plateau phase of the action potential.*

SUMMARY.

1. Insulin hyperpolarizes. It increases the electrical potential difference across cell membranes of cells whose response to insulin is to stimulate glucose transport.

2. Insulin-induced hyperpolarization is probably a step in the transduction chain leading to stimulated glucose transport. IIH precedes stimulated glucose transport. Electrically-produced hyperpolarization increases stereospecific glucose transport in rat muscle.

3. IIH in rat skeletal muscle is caused immediately by decreased ratio of P_{Na}/P_K, with absolute decrease in both P's, and with the major effect on P_{Na}. Therefore, insulin-induced changes in P_{Na} and P_K are also steps in the transduction chain.

4. Insulin increases whole-cell current through a Na^+-conductance dependent early transient K^+ channel. This action has no obvious relationship to the insulin effect on resting P_{Na} and P_K. It appears to concern initiation of repolarization of the action potential, and may, therefore be important in heart muscle and in skeletal muscle.

5. Subsequent to the Symposium, we demonstrated that there is a late, long-lasting inward Ca^{2+} current responsible for the plateau phase of the myoball action potential, and that this current is reduced dramatically by insulin.

ACKNOWLEDGEMENTS

Recent and current studies reported here were
supported by NSF grant DCB-8309232 and NIH grant DK
17574.

REFERENCES

1.Cheng, K., Groarke, J., Ostimehin, B., Haspel,
   H.C., and Sonenberg, M. (1981): *J. Biol.
   Chem.*, 256:649-655.
2.Davis, R.J., Brand, M.D., and Martin, B.R. (1981):
   Biochem. J., 196:133-147.
3.DeMello, W.C. (1967): *Life Sci.*, 6:959-963.
4.Flatman, J.A., and Clausen, T. (1979): *Nature*
   London, 281:580-581.
5.LaManna, V.R., and Ferrier, G.R. (1981): *Am. J.
   Physiol.*, 240(Heart Circ.Physiol.9):H636-H644.
6.Lantz, R.C., Elsas, L.J., and DeHaan, R.L. (1980):
   Proc. Natl. Acad. Sci. USA, 77:3062-3066.
7.Moore, R.D., and Rabovsky, J.L. (1979): *Am. J.
   Physiol.*, 236(Cell Physiol.5):C249-C254.
8.Otsuka, M., and Ohtsuki, I. (1965): *Nature* London,
   207:300-301.
9.Petrozzo, P., and Zierler, K. (1976): *Fed. Proc.*,
   35:602.
10.Wu, F.-S., and Zierler, K. (1986): *Fed. Proc.*,
   45:1009.
11.Wu, F.-S., and Zierler, K. (1987): *Fed. Proc.*,
   46:1279.
12.Zemkova, H., Teisinger, J., and Vyskocil, F.
   (1982): *Biochim. Biophys. Acta*, 720:405-410.
13.Zierler, K.L. (1957): *Science*, 126:1067-1068.
14.Zierler, K.L. (1959): *Am. J. Physiol.*, 197:515-
   523.
15.Zierler, K.L., Rogus, E., and Hazlewood, C.F.
   (1966): *J. Gen. Physiol.*, 49:433-456.
16.Zierler, K., and Rogus, E.M. (1972): *Am. J.
   Physiol.*, 239:E21-E29.
17.Zierler, K., and Rogus, E.M. (1980): *Am. J.
   Physiol.*, 239(Endocrinol.Metab.2):E21-E29.
18.Zierler, K., and Rogus, E.M. (1981): *Am. J.
   Physiol.*, 241(Cell Physiol.10):C145-C149.
19.Zierler, K., and Rogus, E.M. (1981): *Biochim.
   Biophys. Acta*, 640:687-692.
20.Zierler, K., Rogus, E.M., Scherer, R.W., and Wu,
   F.-S. (1985): *Am. J. Physiol.*, 249
   (Endocrinol.Metab.12):E17-E25.
21.Zierler, K., and Wu, F.-S. (1986): *Clinical
   Research*, 34:727A.

Insulin Action and Diabetes,
edited by H. Joseph Goren et al.
Raven Press, New York © 1988.

MEDIATORS OF INSULIN ACTION

Leonard Jarett, M.D.

Department of Pathology and Laboratory Medicine
University of Pennsylvania School of Medicine
3400 Spruce Street
Philadelphia, Pennsylvania 19104

Insulin causes pleiotropic effects in target cells, probably brought about by multiple independent mechanisms. In terms of their time courses, these effects may be observed in milliseconds (ion flux), seconds to minutes (e.g. glucose transport, regulation of carbohydrate and lipid metabolism), or in tens of minutes to hours (regulation of gene expression). With respect to the mechanisms whereby insulin causes these effects, it is evident that the activation of tyrosine kinase probably plays a key proximal role, although the exact nature of this role is not yet clear. For some of the effects of insulin there may also be a role for activated internalized receptor kinase, as described in the talk by Dr. Posner. In addition there appears to be a role for low molecular weight mediators of insulin action. Since the 1970's our own work has focussed on the nature of these mediators.

Early work by Larner's group (9) indicated that extracts of insulin-treated rabbit skeletal muscle (containing a material called factor X) could activate glycogen synthase and inhibit cyclic AMP-dependent protein kinase. Our own work (2, for a review) led to the identification of low molecular weight material present in the supernatant of insulin-treated adipocyte membranes that could activate mitochondrial pyruvate dehydrogenase by dephosphorylation, in a manner that mimicked insulin's effect. Since those early experiments, work from a number of laboratories, including our own, has indicated that there are a number of sources of mediator substances that can mimic the effects of insulin on a variety of enzyme systems. Membranes from tissues as diverse as fat, liver, and human placenta have been shown to yield mediator material (2). Intact cells like hepatocytes, adipocytes, hepatoma cells and human monocytes have also proved to be a source of mediator material (2). In all of these systems, insulin-treated cells yielded more mediator than did control cells. In studies with intact cells, the IM-9 lymphocyte has been an interesting control. This cell, which possesses an insulin-activated tyrosine kinase, has yet to be shown to have a biological response to insulin. In contrast to the other mediator-yielding cells, the IM-9 lymphocyte, when treated with insulin, yielded decreased amounts of pyruvate dehydrogenase (PDH) activating material and increased amounts of a PDH inhibitor (2). Intact animal tissue, as mentioned above, was the first to be shown to be a source of insulin mediator. The early work of Larner and coworkers used insulin-treated rabbits from which mediator was obtained from muscle extracts. Subsequently, we have been able to obtain mediator material from the liver, skeletal muscle and heart of insulin-treated rats. In summary, one can obtain mediator material not only from subcellular systems but also from intact cells and intact tissues in vivo.

The enzyme systems and metabolic processes that have been shown to respond to mediator materials are summarized in Table 1.

TABLE 1:   Enzymes and Metabolic Processes Effected by Insulin Mediators

    A.   Enzymes
        *1.   Pyruvate dehydrogenase
        *2.   Glycogen synthase
         3.   cAMP dependent protein kinase
         4.   Low Km cyclic AMP phosphodiesterase
         5.   Adenylate cyclase
         6.   Acetyl-Co A decarboxylase
         7.   Glucose-6-phosphatase
        *8.   Phospholipid methyltransferase

    *whole cell assay as well as in vitro

    B.   Metabolic Processes
         1.   Lipogenesis
         2.   Antilipolysis
         3.   Lowering of cAMP
         4.   Glucose transport (no effect)

The regulation of all of these enzymes or metabolic processes would appear to involve principally, the regulation of phosphorylation. A variety of investigators have demonstrated effects of putative mediators of insulin action in such enzyme systems (2). In addition to regulating isolated enzyme systems, mediator materials have been shown to affect enzyme activity (PDH, glycogen synthase, phospholipid methyltransferase) in intact adipocytes (4,5,6). Mediator material has also been observed, like insulin, to stimulate lipogenesis, to inhibit hormone-stimulated lipolysis and to lower cyclic AMP levels in intact cells (1,13). The one action that we have not been able to mimic with the mediators is the direct stimulation of glucose transport in adipocytes (5), indicating that the mediators do not account for all of insulin's actions and that multiple mechanisms must exist to account for insulin's pleiotropic effects. In summary, one can state that our work over a period of about eight years has established that insulin generates a low-molecular-weight acid- and heat-stable material from subcellular, whole cell systems and from intact animals that can mimic the action of insulin on insulin-sensitive enzymes and metabolic pathways, both in vitro and in vivo.

The exact chemical identity of the mediator material has yet to be determined. Our laboratory has, for some time, been involved in attempts to characterize this material. Although originally, the mediator material appeared to be a single polypeptide, but that was soon disproved. More recent data indicate that the material is lipid in nature as first suggested by our laboratory (3). Work by Saltiel and coworkers (12) has made a major contribution in this area, suggesting that the material is a novel glycolipid, containing glucosamine, inositol and phosphate. Our recent work has followed this lead, focussing on material that we believe might represent the precursor of the mediator. We sought to purify the precursor, which should yield mediator as a product via the action of phospholipase C. It is hypothesized that, similar to the anchoring system of trypanosomes, a unique phospholipase C will release an inositol-containing glycan which would act as a mediator for insulin action. We have used radioactive glucosamine to label H35 hepatoma cells in an attempt to isolate the precursor material (10). From such glucosamine-labeled cells it has proved possible to isolate, by extraction and thin layer chromatography, a radioactive glucosamine-containing glycophospholipid. Our data showed that after treating H35 cells with insulin, there is a dramatic decrease in the amount of this material that can be recovered from the cells.

In an attempt to determine the other compounds linked to the insulin sensitive glycophospholipid along with glucosamine, we prelabeled the H35 cells with a variety of other compounds (sorbitol, ethanolamine, serine and inositol); using glucosamine as 100%, we found virtually no incorporation of any of these compounds into the fraction that simultaneously contained glucosamine. We were concerned because of the lack of our ability to detect incorporated inositol, in view of the findings of Saltiel and coworkers (12). Because of previous difficulties outlined in the trypanosome literature relating to the detection of incorporated inositol, we chose an alternative means to determine whether or not inositol was present in our glucosamine-containing compound. The approach we used involved labeling the precursor in H35 hepatoma cells with both radioactive glucosamine and palmitate. Palmitate was found to be incorporated 10 fold more than myristate. In our isolation procedure, glucosamine-and palmitate-containing compounds co-migrated. By treating the glucosamine-containing phospholipid with nitrous acid, the glucosamine was released leaving us with a labeled mixture migrating in the position of phosphatidylinositol, suggesting that indeed inositol was present (10). Following this experiment we labeled cells with ^{32}P and used the same approach, first treating the isolated glucosamine-containing material with nitrous acid and then treating the released material, presumed to be phosphatidylinositol, with phospholipase C. Upon high pressure chromatography of the water-soluble material released by phospholipase C, we observed that more than 90% of the material eluted in the position of the inositol phosphate standard (11). We therefore felt confident that the glucosamine-containing glycophospholipid also contained inositol.

Upon treating the isolated lipid with phospholipase A_2, the palmitate label was found to be both in the neutral lipid fraction and in the lyso-compound. Thus, palmitate appeared to be at both positions one and two of the phospholipid. Interestingly, when we treated the material with PI-specific phospholipase C (supplied to us by Dr. Martin Low), we were surprised to find that the precursor did not yield diacylglycerol, but 1 akyl, 2 acyl glycerol. These data suggested to us that the radioactivity from palmitate might be incorporated via an ether linkage at position 1 rather than via an ester bond. We do not know the physiological meaning of these results at present. Our recent work suggests that there are at least two additional phosphate moieties in the compound and that the inositol may be the chiro form and that four galactoses are present (11). In addition, the glucosamine was determined to be galactosamine by GC/mass spectroscopy (11).

After treating the glycosamine-containing glycophospholipid material with phospholipase C, the water soluble component was eluted from a P2 column in the same position that we detected the biological activity as discussed below. So, in summary, we believe we have in our hands a compound that looks as follows:

1 akyl, 2 acyl glycerol (dipalmitate)
|
phosphate
|
inositol (chiro)
|
galactosamine
|
galactose (4)
|
phosphate (2)

Isolation of mediator from tissues is complicated by the fact that the compound, depending on the source and techniques of extraction, can interact with Mg^+ and Ca^+, thereby altering chromatographic characteristics and thereby making isolation difficult (Gottschalk and Jarett, submitted). The phospho- oligosaccharide generated from the glycophospholipid precursor also complexed with cations when added to muscle or liver extract, rendering it cationic when it is anionic in its native state. This ability of the mediator to complex cations may be important to the mediator action on pyruvate dehydrogenase.

The material from the H35 hepatoma cells works in intact adipocytes to block lipolysis in a manner that mimics the effect of 100 microunits/ml of insulin (8). In addition, the mediator from H35 cells works both in an intact cell and at the subcellular level to stimulate pyruvate dehydrogenase (Gottschalk and Jarett, submitted) and to inhibit phospholipid methyltransferase (7). As with our previous work with mediator material, the substance from H35 cells does not stimulate glucose transport (as reflected by increased glucose oxidation) in an adipocyte preparation where insulin causes marked stimulation.

In summary, we believe we have a good lead on the structure of the putative mediator material from H35 cells.   From the work that we have done over a number of years I am convinced that the mediator materials from different cells will turn out to be members of a new family of compounds. In support of this concept, we have obtained material from at least three different cell types in which we can introduce a radioactive label but with slightly different properties.

In summary, a simplistic scheme of insulin action would portray the activation of tyrosine kinase by insulin as an initial event triggering insulin action.   This enzyme activation may bring about, via the phosphorylation of target proteins (possibly a G protein of some type), the activation of a unique phospholipase C.   The identity of the specific phospholipase C which is present in plasma membranes from liver, H35 cells and adipocytes remains to be determined.   In terms of our own work, we would postulate that the activated phospholipase C acts on the glycophospholipid we have detected in our H35 extracts,   releasing   a   phospho-oligosaccharide mediator akin to the compound(s) observed by Saltiel and coworkers (12).   Clearly, much more work remains to be done on what may turn out to be a family of glycophospholipid precursors that yield phospho-oligosaccharide mediators which regulate enzymes that are the targets for insulin action.   It is my conviction that these small molecular weight molecules that are generated from the plasma membrane, will be found to play a key role in the short term intracellular actions of insulin.

Acknowledgements

This work was supported by NIH grant AM28144. The work reported from this laboratory was generated by my colleagues: Andy Abler, Kirby Gottschalk, Kathleen Kelly, Janet Macaulay, Lance Macaulay, and Jose Mato.

References

1. Caro, J.R., Folli, F., Cacchin, F., and Sinha, M.K. (1983):   Biochim. Biophys. Res. Commun., 115:375-382.
2. Gottschalk, W.K., Macaulay, S.L., Macaulay, J.O., Kelly, K., Smith, J.A., and Jarett, L.   (1986): In: Annals of the New York Academy of Sciences: Membrane Pathology, pp. 385-405; Gottschalk, W.K. and Jarett, L. (1985): In: Diabetes/Metabolism Reviews, John Wiley and Sons, Inc.

3. Jarett, L., Kiechle, F.L., and Parker, J.C. (1982): Fed. Proc., 41:2736-2741.
4. Jarett, L., Macaulay, S.L., Macaulay, J.O., Kelly, K.A., Wong, E.H.A., Smith, J.A., and Gottschalk, K. (1986): In: Diabetes, edited by M. Serrano Rios and P.J. Lefibore, pp. 89-93, Excerpta Medica, Amsterdam-New York-Oxford.
5. Jarett, L., Wong, E.H.A., and Smith, J.A. (1985): Science, 227:533-539.
6. Jarett, L., Wong, E.H.A., Smith, J.A., and Macaulay, S.L. (1985): Endocrinology, 116:1011-1016.
7. Kelly, K.L., Mato, J.M., and Jarett, L. (1986): FEBS, 209:238-242.
8. Kelly, K.L., Mato, J.M., Merida, I., and Jarett, L. (1987): Proc. Natl. Acad. Sci., 84:6404-6407.
9. Larner, J., Takeda, Y., Brewer, H.B., Brooker, G., and Murad, F. (1976): In: Metabolic Interconversions of Enzymes, edited by S. Shatiel. Springer-Verlag, New York.
10. Mato, J.M., Kelly, K.L., Abler, A., and Jarett, L. (1987): J. Biol. Chem., 262:2131-2137.
11. Mato, J.M., Kelly, K.L., Abler, A., Jarett, L., Corkey, B.E., Cashel, J.A., and Zopf, D. (1987): Biochem. Biophys. Res. Comm., 146:764-770.
12. Saltiel, A., and Cuatrecasas, P. (1986): Proc. Natl. Acad. Sci., 83:5793-5797; Saltiel, A., Fox, J.A., Sherline, P., and Cuatrecasas, P. (1986): Science, 233:967-972.
13. Zhang, S.-R., Shi, G.-H., and Ho., R. (1983): J. Biol. Chem., 258:6471-6476.

Insulin Action and Diabetes,
edited by H. Joseph Goren et al.
Raven Press, New York © 1988.

MECHANISM OF PHOSPHOLIPASE C ACTIVATION BY INSULIN

IN RAT ADIPOCYTES

Jose Goldman, and Benjamin A. Rybicki

Henry Ford Hospital
2799 West Grand Boulevard
Detroit, Michigan, U.S.A. 48202

Insulin activates phospholipase C (PLC) in rat adipocytes (2, 3,6). This activation closely correlates with the stimulation of adipocyte hexose transport rates with regard to both time dependence and insulin dose-response relationships. Thus, adipocyte PLC activity rises as early as 1 min and peaks at 3 min after the addition of insulin (100 μU/ml) at 37°C, and both stimulation of hexose transport and PLC activation occur maximally at 100 μU/ml of insulin and have ED_{50} values of 28 μU/ml of insulin (3). The insulin activated PLC has been shown to be a phosphoinositide phosphodiesterase predominantly localized in the cytoplasmic fraction (4). In order to define the mechanism of adipocyte PLC activation by insulin, we have studied the steady state kinetics of PLC both at basal and insulin stimulated conditions.

METHODS

Male Sprague-Dawley rats were obtained from Charles River Laboratories (Wilmington, MA). Rat adipocytes were isolated as described by Rodbell (10). Adipocytes ($2\text{-}4\times10^5$ cells/ml) were incubated at 37°C in 25 mM Hepes, 25 mM Tricine, buffer pH 7.4 containing 110 mM NaCl, 3.5 mM KCl, 1.2 mM $MgCl_2$, 2.5 mM $CaCl_2$ and 1% BSA with and without insulin (100 μU/ml) to activate PLC maximally (average time: 3 min). At the end of the incubation, aliquots of the cell suspension were sonicated at 4°C for 20 sec, and the fat layer was removed after centrifugation. Resonication as before produced homogenates. Protein concentration was determined by the method of Lowry et al. (8). PLC assays were performed using a modification of the procedure of Koepfer-Hobelsberger and Wieland (6) as follows: incubations were performed in Tris-maleate buffer pH 7.5 with (^{3}H)phosphatidyl inositol as substrate (0.05 μCi/ml, 0.05 to 1.0 mM) at 37°C for 3 min. Because this time is within the limits of linearity, the measured enzyme activities represent initial velocities. Assay sample volumes varied from 10 to 50 µl. At the end of the incubation period, incubates were extracted with aliquots of chloroform: methanol (2:1, v/v). After centrifugation at 4°C for 1 min, aliquots of the aqueous phase were counted in a liquid scintillation spectrometer. Nonenzymatic substrate hydrolysis was corrected for with incubations omitting the homogenates.

RESULTS AND DISCUSSION

Results of four independent experiments were averaged and analyzed by means of the linearized equation $v = (Vmax) - (Km)(v/S)$ (Eadie-Hofstee plot) (5), where symbols have standard meanings. Apparent Vmax and Km values were calculated from the ordinate and abscissa intercepts, respectively, and they are given in the following table.

Effect of insulin on the kinetic parameters of rat adipocyte phospholipase C

	Km (mM)	Vmax (nmoles.min^{-1}.mg $protein^{-1}$)
Control	0.91	68.14
Insulin	1.59	131.94

The data indicate that insulin activates rat adipocyte PLC through a two-fold increase in Vmax with no change in Km. Although the structural and/or conformational alterations in the PLC molecule that underlie the change in enzyme Vmax brought about by insulin remain to be determined, considerable experimental evidence supports a role for these biochemical events in the mechanism of insulin stimulation of hexose transport and other insulin effects. Insulin produces an early stimulation of the synthesis of inositol phosphates (IP, IP2 and IP3) (2) and diacylglycerol (DAG) (1) which are products of phosphoinositide hydrolysis by PLC. DAG is an activator of protein kinase C (9), and the phorbol ester activation of this enzyme also leads to effects similar to those of insulin (1,7,11). In conclusion, insulin activation of adipocyte PLC through an increase in enzyme Vmax is related to the stimulation of hexose transport.

REFERENCES

1. Farese, R.V., Davis, J.S., Barnes, D.E., Standaert, M.L. and Pollet, R.J. (1984): *J. Biol. Chem.*, 259:7094-7100.
2. Farese, R.V., Kuo, J.Y., Babischkin, J.S., and Davis, J.S. (1986): *J. Biol. Chem.*, 261:8589-8592.
3. Goldman, J., and Rybicki, B.A. (1986): *Diabetes*, 35:320.

4.   Goldman, J. and Rybicki, B.A. (1987): *Diabetes*, 36:52.
5.   Hofstee, B.H.J. (1952): *J. Biol. Chem.*, 199:357-364.
6.   Koepfer-Hobelsberger, B. and Wieland, O. (1984): *Mol. Cell. Endocrinol.*, 36:123-129.
7.   Lee, L.-S. and Weinstein, I.B. (1979): *J. Cell. Physiol.*, 99:451-460.
8.   Lowry, O.H., Rosebrough, N.J., Farr, A.L. and Randall, R.J. (1951): *J. Biol. Chem.*, 193:265-275.
9.   Nishizuka, Y. (1984): *Nature*, 308:693-698.
10.   Rodbell, M.J. (1964): *J. Biol. Chem.*, 239:375-380.
11.   Van de Werve, G., Proietto, J. and Jeanrenaud, B. (1985): *Biochem. J.*, 225:523-527.

Financial support by the R.W. Smith - W.H. Searight Diabetes Research Fund is gratefully acknowledged.

Insulin Action and Diabetes,
edited by H. Joseph Goren et al.
Raven Press, New York © 1988.

IDENTIFICATION AND ROLE OF A 15-KILODALTON CELLULAR TARGET OF THE INSULIN RECEPTOR TYROSINE KINASE

Michel Bernier, Don M. Laird and M. Daniel Lane

Department of Biological Chemistry
The Johns Hopkins University School of Medicine
Baltimore, Maryland 21205, USA

The insulin receptor is a transmembrane allosteric enzyme which possesses both a cell surface hormone (activator) binding site and a cytoplasmic tyrosine kinase catalytic site (9). These functional domains are covalently linked through a transmembrane stretch of hydrophobic amino acid residues (4,9,12). Studies with cell-free receptor preparations indicate that the interaction of insulin with its specific binding site activates tyrosine kinase function at the remote catalytic site. Initially autophosphorylation of the receptor itself occurs followed by phosphorylation of model substrates, such as histone, casein and reduced and carboxyamidomethylated lysozyme. Despite numerous attempts the identification of bonafide cellular targets of the insulin receptor kinase with defined function has remained elusive.

RELATIONSHIP OF INSULIN RECEPTOR ACTION TO STIMULATION OF HEXOSE UPTAKE

This report will focus on the characteristics of a 15-kilodalton cytoplasmic protein discovered recently in this laboratory (1) that we believe to be a physiological target of the insulin receptor kinase in mouse adipocytes. We have used the fully differentiated 3T3-L1 adipocyte as a model cell system. These cells differentiate in culture into cells that have the morphological and biochemical characteristics of adipocytes; thus, they acquire pleiotropic responsiveness to insulin. In our work the biological response that has served as the indicator of insulin action is insulin-activated hexose uptake. As shown in Fig. 1 the basal rate of hexose uptake by 3T3-L1 adipocytes without insulin present is slow and linear for 10 min. If insulin is added, after a short lag, there is an increase of about ten-fold in the rate of hexose uptake.
Several years ago we observed (6) that when the trivalent

117

arsenical (phenylarsineoxide) was added, either before or at the time of insulin addition, the insulin-activated component of hexose uptake was totally blocked (Fig. 1).

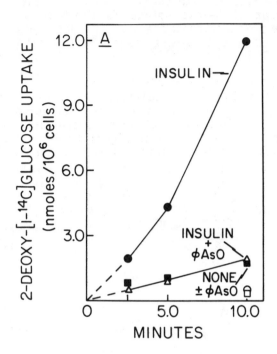

FIG. 1.   Activation of hexose uptake by insulin and its inhibition by phenylarsineoxide in 3T3-L1 adipocytes. 2-deoxy[1-^{14}C]-glucose (0.2 mM) uptake was measured over a 10- minute period in the presence or absence of 1 μM insulin in cells pretreated or not with 35 μM phenylarsineoxide. Some cell monolayers were pretreated for 10 minutes with cytochalasin B (20 μM) and then assayed for hexose uptake with (0) or without ($\square$) insulin as above. Half-maximal transport activation is achieved at 7 nM insulin. The results are from Frost and Lane (6).

Phenylarsineoxide has an interesting chemistry in biological systems since it interacts rather specifically with vicinal or neighboring dithiols (6). Dithiols of this type form relatively stable ring complexes with phenylarsineoxide, although this reaction can be reversed. An example is the dihydrolipoyl prosthetic group of pyruvate dehydrogenase which is the site of inhibition by arsenite, another trivalent arsenical. This inhibition can be reversed by a vicinal dithiol competitor such as 2,3-dimercaptopropanol, but not by monothiols. When 3T3-L1 adipocytes are treated with phenylarsineoxide, the insulin-stimulated component of hexose uptake is blocked, but there is no effect on the basal component (Fig. 1). Both basal and insulin-stimulated hexose uptake are nearly completely inhibited by cytochalasin B indicating involvement of the classical glucose transporter.

Our results with the trivalent arsenical, led us to believe that a vicinal dithiol intermediate(s) is involved in the signal transmission pathway between the insulin receptor and the glucose transport system (Fig. 2A). Evidence supporting the hypothesis that phenylarsineoxide interrupts signal transmission by complexing this putative dithiol intermediate (X-tyr-P; Fig. 2A) is presented below.

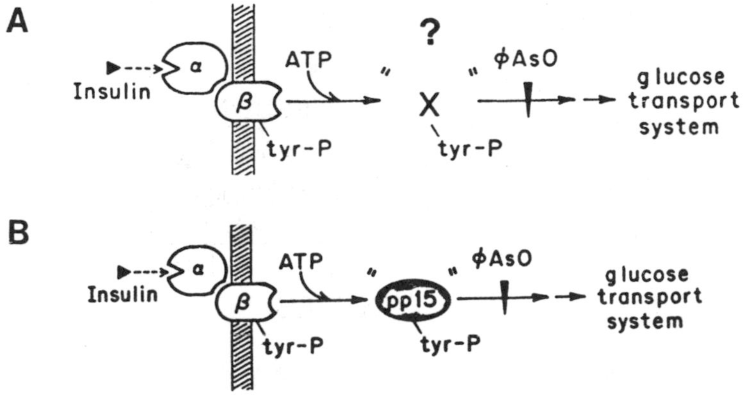

A

Insulin ----▷ α β ATP ? φAsO → X → glucose transport system

tyr-P tyr-P

B

Insulin ----▷ α β ATP φAsO → (pp15) → glucose transport system

tyr-P tyr-P

FIG. 2.   Possible effect of phenylarsineoxide on the insulin-activated signal transmission pathway. A) Pathway showing X-tyr-P as an hypothetical intermediate. B) Pathway showing pp15-tyr-P as an intermediate. The results are from Bernier et. al. (1).

To ascertain the kinetic relationship between the activation of autophosphorylation of the β-subunit of the receptor by insulin and the onset of the activation of glucose uptake, the progress of both of these events was monitored following stimulation of 3T3-L1 adipocytes with insulin (7). 3T3-L1 adipocytes were first incubated for 2 hours with inorganic phosphate labeled with ^{32}P. We have established (7) that within 2 hours the specific activities of the α, β, and γ phosphoryl groups of ATP reach a constant level. Insulin was added and then at various time intervals thereafter the cells were lysed with sodium dodecylsulfate to prevent any further phosphorylation or dephosphorylation and to extract the insulin receptor. The α and β subunits of the receptor were then isolated and resolved and ^{32}P-activity incorporated into the β-subunit was determined.

Concomitantly, experiments were conducted in which [^{14}C] 3-0-methylglucose uptake rates were measured at intervals to assess the correspondence between β-subunit phosphorylation and the activation of hexose uptake (7).

   As shown in Fig. 3, some ^{32}P-activity is associated with the receptor's β-subunit even before insulin is added. We have

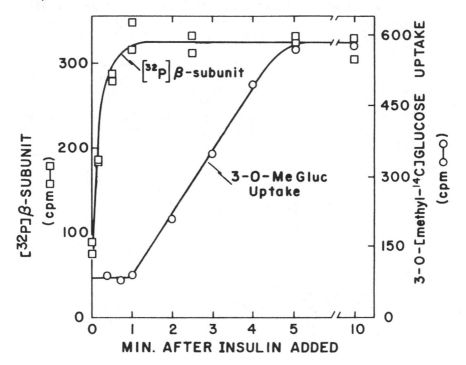

FIG.3.   Comparison of insulin receptor β-subunit phosphorylation and 3-0-methylglucose uptake rate following stimulation by insulin. 3T3-L1 adipocytes were exposed to 1 μM insulin for time periods indicated. The uptake of 3-0-[methyl-^{14}C]glucose was measured for a 20-sec period after the indicated periods of time following the addition of insulin. To determine the extent of phosphorylation of the insulin receptor β-subunit, cells were exposed to medium containing ^{32}P for 2 hours to label the ATP pool to constant ^{32}P specific activity (7). At various times after exposing the cells to insulin further phosphorylation or dephosphorylation was halted by the addition of 0.1% SDS. This was followed by dilution with 1% Triton-X-100 and adsorbing the receptor quantitatively to wheat-germ lectin Sepharose and elution with N-acetylglucosamine. ^{32}P-labeled β-subunit was then isolated by 2-dimensional SDS polyacrylamide gel electrophoresis. Radioactivity associated with the β-subunit was quantitated by cutting out the gel spot and counting. The results are from Kohanski et. al. (7).

established that this is due primarily to serine phosphate (7), and there is virtually no phosphotyrosine at this point. After addition of insulin, however, rapid ^{32}P-phosphorylation of the receptor occurs and this increment is almost exclusively in phosphotyrosine (7). The receptor achieves ($t_{1/2} \cong$ 10 seconds) and maintains a steady-state level of phosphorylation for at least 10 minutes. As shown in Fig. 3 basal hexose uptake is maintained for about 60 seconds after insulin addition and then begins to rise. The rate increases, but does not achieve maximal rate until about 4 to 5 minutes. Following this lag, the rate remains constant for at least 10 minutes. These results indicate that there is rapid insulin-stimulated phosphorylation (apparently autophosphorylation) of the receptor on tyrosine which we presume to be involved in the signal transmission process. Following rapid phosphorylation of the receptor there is a much slower onset of activation of hexose uptake.

INDENTIFICATION AND CHARACTERIZATION OF A PHOSPHOTYROSYL PROTEIN TARGET, pp15, OF THE INSULIN RECEPTOR KINASE

Based upon the results described above and upon other findings which indicate that insulin receptor function per se is not affected by phenylarsineoxide (5), the minimal sequence of events in the signal transmission pathway, illustrated in Fig. 2A, was formulated. It is established that insulin activates receptor autophosphorylation, and thereby, the receptor's tyrosine protein kinase activity (8, 10). The receptor kinase then catalyzes phosphorylation (on tyrosine) of the cellular protein substrate, i.e. X-tyr-P, a putative intermediate in the pathway controlling hexose uptake. It was proposed (6) and recently verified (1,5) that phenylarsineoxide blocks insulin-activated hexose uptake at a point beyond the insulin receptor tyrosine kinase.

After a number of unsuccessful attempts to demonstrate insulin-activated tyrosine phosphorylation of a cellular target in situ in 3T3-L1 adipocytes a new strategy was developed (1). The possibility was considered that the ^{32}P-labeled phosphoryl group (on tyrosine) of the putative cellular substrate turned over too rapidly to detect. Phenylarsineoxide, which appeared to act down-stream from the receptor, might block this turnover and cause the accumulation of the phosphorylated intermediate. This approach proved successful (1). The protocol to test this hypothesis involved: preliminary incubation of 3T3-L1 adipocytes with inorganic ^{32}P-orthophosphate for 2 hours, then the addition (or not) of phenylarsineoxide, followed by the addition (or not) of insulin. Ten minutes after the addition of insulin, the reaction was quenched and cell extracts were analyzed by 2-dimensional isoelectric focusing/SDS gel electrophoresis. As shown in Fig. 4D a phosphorylated 15 kDa protein with a pI of about 6.3 accumulated when the cells were treated with both insulin and phenylarsineoxide, but not in the absence of either or both insulin and phenylarsineoxide (Fig. 4A, B and C). Phosphoamino acid analysis performed on the ^{32}P-labeled 15-kDa protein,

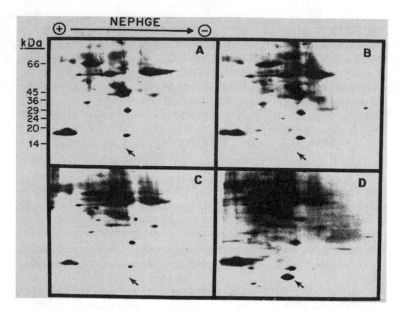

FIG. 4.   Insulin- and phenylarsineoxide-dependent accumulation of a phosphorylated 15 kDa polypeptide, pp15, in 3T3-L1 adipocytes.   Cell monolayers were labeled for 2 hours with $^{32}P_i$-containing medium.   This was followed by a 10-min preincubation without (A, B) or with (C, D) phenylarsineoxide (35 µM) and then a 10-min incubation without (A, C) or with (B, D) insulin (1 µM). Cells were lysed in urea-containing sample buffer and phosphorylated proteins were analyzed by 2-dimensional gel electrophoresis with non-equilibrium isoelectric focusing (NEPHGE) in the first dimension and SDS/polyacrylamide gel electrophoresis in the second dimension.   Equal amounts of cell extract were loaded onto gels. ^{32}P-labeled proteins were detected by autoradiography. The results are from Bernier et. al. (1).

henceforth referred to as pp15, revealed that phosphorylation occurred exclusively on tyrosine (1).   Thus, the hypothesis that insulin activates phosphorylation of a cellular protein via the insulin receptor kinase and that phenylarsineoxide blocks the turnover of this phosphotyrosyl protein intermediate, i.e. pp15, appears to be correct (see Fig. 2B).

We then set out to further characterize the processes by which pp15 is formed and which lead to its accumulation.   To assess the role of the insulin receptor kinase in the phosphorylation of p15 (or its precursor) the insulin concentration dependence, and the kinetics and hormone ligand specificity of β-subunit phosphorylation and of pp15 formation were compared.   It was found (1) that both phosphorylation processes exhibit identical insulin concentration dependences, i.e. both are activated to the same extent and exhibit similar K_A's.   Furthermore, whereas pp15 accumulation is absolutely dependent upon the presence of phenylarsineoxide, phosphorylation of the insulin receptor's β-subunit is unaffected by the arsenical. These findings are consistent with the hypothesis (see Fig. 2B) that the insulin receptor kinase phosphorylates p15 (or its precursor) and that phenylarsineoxide, which prevents the turnover of ^{32}P-pp15, has no measureable effect on the autophosphorylation of the insulin receptor <u>per se</u> (and thus, has no effect on its tyrosine kinase activity).

Kinetic experiments were conducted in which the progress of β-subunit phosphorylation, pp15 accumulation and the activation of hexose uptake were monitored following stimulation of cells by insulin. As illustrated in Fig. 5 the β-subunit of the receptor

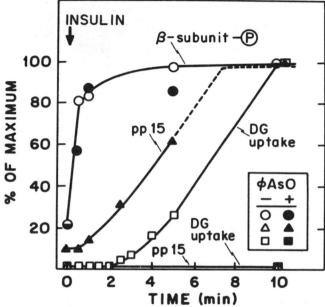

FIG. 5. Comparison of the kinetics of insulin-stimulated insulin receptor β-subunit phosphorylation, pp15 phosphorylation and 2-deoxy-[1-^{14}C]glucose uptake in 3T3-L1 adipocytes. To follow the kinetics of phosphorylation of the insulin receptor's β-subunit and of pp15, cells were first labeled with medium containing ^{32}P$_i$. The cells were then treated (●, ▲) or not (o, Δ) with phenylarsine oxide for 10 minutes followed by insulin addition. The kinetics of 2-deoxy-[1-^{14}C]glucose uptake were determined in cells previously treated (■) or not (□) with 35 μM phenylarsine oxide and stimulated with 1 μM insulin. The maximal level of [^{32}P]labeled β-subunit in the insulin-stimulated steady-state was 542 c.p.m. per 10^6 cells and the maximal level of [^{32}P]pp15 was 601 c.p.m. per 10^6 cells. [^{14}C]2-Deoxyglucose uptake is expressed as insulin-stimulated uptake, corrected for basal uptake, at each time point. Maximal uptake at 10 min was 11.5 nmoles per 10^6 cells. β-Subunit-P refers to [^{32}P]labeled insulin receptor β-subunit and DG refers to [^{14}C]2-deoxyglucose. Results are from Bernier <u>et. al.</u> (1).

is rapidly phosphorylated, followed by the build-up of pp15 (only in the presence of phenylarsineoxide) and somewhat later by the insulin-stimulated increase in hexose uptake. There was a lag of 4-5 minutes which occurred before a linear rate of sugar uptake was achieved. This sequence of these events is consistent with β-subunit phosphorylation occurring first, then phosphorylation of pp15 and finally, the activation of sugar uptake.

A further indication that the insulin receptor kinase is responsible for the phosphorylation of p15 (or its precursor) derives from the hormone/growth factor specificity of the process. The accumulation of pp15 occurs only with insulin. IGF-1, IGF-2, EGF or PDGF, each of which has its own receptor in 3T3-L1 adipocytes, does not activate the accumulation of pp15 (1). It should be noted that, like the insulin receptor, the receptors for IGF-1, EGF and PDGF possess tyrosine kinase activity and undergo ligand-activated autophosphorylation.

There is, in fact, another agent that mimics insulin both with respect to the activation of hexose uptake and formation of pp15 (results not shown). This agent is vanadate. Exposure of 3T3-L1 adipocytes to 1 mM vanadate for 6 hours or longer activates hexose uptake to the same maximal extent of stimulation as with insulin. Moreover, vanadate (in the absence of insulin) induces receptor β-subunit phosphorylation as does insulin. Like insulin alone, however, vanadate does not cause cellular accumulation of pp15. When phenylarsineoxide was added to vanadate-treated cells, pp15 accumulated to the same extent as with insulin plus phenylarsineoxide. Thus, it appears that vanadate, a potent inhibitor of phosphotyrosyl-protein phosphatases, blocks dephosphorylation of the insulin receptor. This action would be expected to increase receptor tyrosine kinase activity and would cause increased phosphorylation of p15 (see Fig. 2B).

ROLE OF pp15 AS AN INTERMEDIATE IN INSULIN-STIMULATED SIGNALLING OF THE GLUCOSE TRANSPORT SYSTEM

Since most regulatory covalent modifications of proteins are "reversible" processes, eg. the phosphorylation/dephosphorylation of many regulatory enzymes, it became important to know whether and, if so how rapidly, the phenylarsineoxide-induced increase in pp15 level could be reversed. To accomplish this, we made use of 2,3-dimercaptopropanol, a vicinal dithiol agent which is capable of complexing trivalent arsenicals, such as phenylarsineoxide (see above and references 1 and 6). As shown above (Fig. 1) inhibition of insulin-stimulated hexose uptake is reversed by the subsequent addition of 2,3-dimercaptopropanol, while a monothiol, eg. 2-mercaptoethanol, is ineffective. The effectiveness of the vicinal dithiol, 2,3-dimercaptopropanol, in reversing the phenyl-arsineoxide-/insulin-induced cellular accumulation of pp15 is demonstrated in Fig. 6. Thus, following addition of the dithiol, there is a rapid fall in pp15 level, i.e. an 80% drop within 1 min (2). The monothiol, 2-mercaptoethanol, has no effect (results not shown). It is evident, therefore, that by "removing"

phenylarsineoxide with a dithiol agent the blockade is reversed
and the phosphoryl group of pp15 turns over rapidly. This
finding provides an explanation for why pp15 does not accumulate
when cells are treated with insulin alone and lends further
support to the sequence of events proposed in Fig. 2B. Since
insulin activates the phosphorylation (of p15) by its receptor
tyrosine kinase, yet pp15 does not accumulate, we can conclude
that the rate of dephosphorylation of pp15 is considerably faster
than its rate of formation (phosphorylation).

We suspected that the 4-5 minute lag in achieving maximal
glucose uptake rate after insulin addition (See Figs. 3 and 5)
might be due to a slow rate of pp15 formation relative to the
turnover of its phosphoryltyrosine group(s). This hypothesis was
tested (2) by first raising the cellular level of pp15 by
stimulating its formation with insulin, while blocking turnover
with phenylarsineoxide (Fig. 6). Under these conditions the

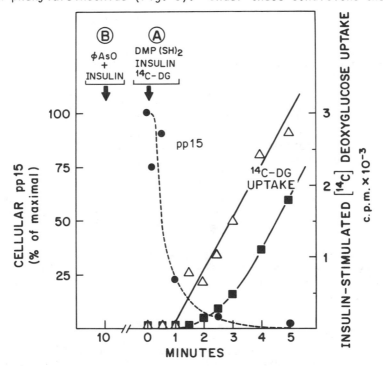

FIG. 6. Effect of 2,3-dimercaptopropanol on the kinetics of
reversal of pp15 accumulation and inhibition of hexose uptake
caused by phenylarsineoxide in the presence of insulin. 3T3-L1
adipocytes (labeled or not with $^{32}P_i$, see Fig. 4) were treated or
not for 10 minutes with phenylarsineoxide and insulin prior to
initiating hexose uptake by the addition of 2,3-dimercaptopro-
panol, insulin and [^{14}C]2-deoxyglucose. ^{14}C-Hexose uptake was
then followed as described in Figure 1 and ^{32}P-pp15 levels
monitored as in Figure 4. Results are from Bernier <u>et. al.</u> (1).

activation of hexose uptake by insulin is blocked, presumably because signal transmission beyond pp15 is interrupted by phenylarsineoxide (see Fig. 2B). Then, the blockade by phenylarsineoxide was rapidly released by the addition of the vicinal dithiol, 2,3-dimercaptopropanol. This resulted in a precipitous fall in the cellular level of pp15 and a sudden increase in hexose uptake rate. Most importantly, this increase in hexose uptake occurred without the usual lag and was linear from the point of its inception (Fig. 6). These results strongly suggest that it is not the cellular level of pp15 per se which causes the activation of hexose uptake, but rather that the turnover of its phosphoryl group (either by dephosphorylation or transphosphorylation to an acceptor molecule) is tightly coupled to the process by which sugar uptake is activated. Although the coupling mechanism is not yet understood, this concept will guide our future studies on its molecular basis.

PRELIMINARY RESULTS AND FUTURE DIRECTIONS

Finally in results not shown, we have determined that ^{32}P-pp15 is localized in the cytosolic fraction of 3T3-L1 adipocytes. Thus, phosphorylated pp15 would be expected to be mobile and capable of translocating from its site of formation at the cytoplasmic face of the plasma membrane (by the tyrosine kinase domain of the β-subunit) to the intracellular membrane site of the glucose transporter. The cytosolic localization of pp15 raises the possibility that this agent may act pleiotropically to mediate other insulin-activated processes.

We have recently identified and isolated from 3T3-L1 adipocytes (K. Liao, M. Bernier and M. D. Lane, unpublished results) a membrane-bound enzyme activity that causes the removal of the phosphoryl group from pp15. This enzymatic activity is inhibited by phenylarsineoxide and the inhibition can be reversed by the vicinal dithiol, 2,3-dimercaptopropanol, but not monothiol. The characterization of this enzyme and its action should prove useful in determining the molecular basis of the coupling of the phosphoryltyrosine (of pp15) turnover to the activation of hexose uptake.

DISCUSSION AND SUMMARY

A large body of evidence indicates that the multiple cellular actions of insulin are initiated by activation of the tyrosine-specific protein kinase of the insulin receptor (9). We have identified a cellular target of the receptor kinase which appears to mediate insulin-stimulated glucose uptake. In intact 3T3-L1 adipocytes, insulin stimulates autophosphorylation of the receptor's β-subunit. This stimulation of β-subunit phosphorylation is due entirely to an increased level of [^{32}P]phosphotyrosine in the receptor. Thus, upon addition of insulin to 3T3-L1 adipocytes, ^{32}P-orthophosphate incorporation into the β-subunit of the insulin receptor on tyrosyl residues is increased 7-fold and is complete within 1 minute ($t_{1/2}$ = 10 seconds). Kinetic experiments with intact 3T3-L1 adipocytes support the hypothesis that β-subunit autophosphorylation is an intermediate step connecting insulin binding to increased hexose transport rate.

Insulin stimulates hexose uptake by approximately 10-fold in the mature 3T3-L1 adipocyte. Following insulin addition there is a 4-5 minute lag period before maximal hexose uptake rate is achieved. Phenylarsineoxide, a trivalent arsenical that forms stable ring complexes with vicinal dithiols, prevents the activation of hexose uptake by insulin in a concentration-dependent manner, but has no inhibitory effect on basal hexose uptake. 2,3-Dimercaptopropanol prevents, or rapidly reverses, the inhibition of hexose uptake, while 2-mercaptoethanol, a monothiol, has no effect. These results suggest that phenylarsineoxide inhibits signal transmission at a point between the receptor and the glucose transport system. Phenylarsineoxide has no effect on insulin receptor function per se.

Insulin activates the phosphorylation of a tyrosyl residue(s) on a 15 kDa cytosolic protein (pp15) which accumulates when 3T3-L1 adipocytes are treated with phenylarsineoxide. Several lines of evidence implicate pp15 in insulin receptor-induced signal transduction to the glucose transport system. The reciprocal effects of phenylarsineoxide on insulin-stimulated accumulation of pp15 and hexose uptake are both reversed by the vicinal dithiol, 2,3-dimercaptopropanol, but not by the monothiol, 2-mercaptoethanol. Thus, a cellular dithiol appears to function in the signal transmission pathway downstream from pp15. Furthermore, both hexose uptake and phenylarsineoxide-dependent pp15 accumulation exhibit identical insulin concentration dependencies. Like insulin-activated autophosphorylation of the receptors' β-subunit (on tyrosine), activation of the phosphorylation of pp15 (or its precursor) is specific, with IGF-1 and 2, EGF and PDGF being inactive. Vanadate, which activates hexose uptake and insulin receptor β-subunit phosphorylation, also causes the accumulation of pp15, but only in the presence of phenylarsineoxide.

Two findings link insulin-stimulated phosphorylation of pp15 to the activation of hexose uptake. First, phenylarsineoxide affects both processes in an inverse manner and these effects are specifically reversed by the vicinal dithiol reagent, 2,3-dimercaptopropanol, but not by a monothiol, 2-mercaptoethanol. This result implicates an essential dithiol intermediate in the signal transmission pathway which interacts with, or downstream from, pp15. Second, kinetic evidence suggests that the formation of pp15 in response to insulin is the rate-limiting step in signal transmission to the glucose transport system and is responsible for the long (5 min) lag in achieving maximal hexose uptake after insulin addition. Thus, by allowing cellular pp15 to accumulate in the presence of insulin and phenylarsineoxide and then quickly releasing the phenylarsineoxide-induced blockade with 2,3-dimercaptopropanol, thereby by-passing the rate-limiting step, eliminates the usual lag in achieving maximal hexose uptake rate.

This result further suggests that dephosphorylation of (or trans-phosphorylation from) pp15 is coupled to signal transmission to the glucose transport system. Taken together the results presented in this paper are consistent with an intermediary signalling role for pp15 in the insulin-stimulated glucose uptake.

REFERENCES

1.   Bernier, M., Laird, D. and Lane, M. D. (1987)
     Proc. Natl.Acad. Sci., USA, 84, 1844-1848.
2.   Bernier, M., Laird, D. and Lane, M.D. (1987) manuscript in preparation.
3.   Cushman, S.W. and Wardzala, L.J. (1980) J. Biol. Chem., 255, 4758-4762.
4.   Ebina, Y., Ellis, L., Jarnagin, K., Edery, M., Graf, L., Clauser, E., Ou, J-H., Masiarz, F., Kan, Y. W., Goldfine, I.D., Roth, R.A. and Rutter, W. J., (1985) Cell, 40, 747-758
5.   Frost, S.C., Kohanski, R.A. and Lane, M.D. (1987) J. Biol. Chem., 262, 9872-9876.
6.   Frost, S.C. and Lane, M. D., (1985) J. Biol. Chem., 260, 2646-2652.
7.   Kohanski, R.A., Frost, S.C., and Lane, M.D., (1986) J. Biol. Chem., 261, 12272-12281.
8.   Kohanski, R.A. and Lane, M.D. (1986) Biochem. Biophys. Res. Communs., 134, 1312-1318.
9.   Lane, M.D. (1985) Life-Cycle and Regulation of the Insulin Receptor, in "Insulin: Its Receptor and Diabetes," M. D. Hollenberg, ed., Marcel Dekker, Inc., New York, pp. 237-264.
10. Lane, M.D., Kohanski, R.A. (1986) Control of autophosphor-ylation and substrate phosphorylation by the insulin receptor protein kinase, in Proceedings of the Eric K. Fernstron Symposium on Mechanisms of Insulin Action, edited by P. Belfrage, J. Donner and P. Stralfors, p. 59-73, Elsevier, Amsterdam.
11. Susuki, K., and Kono, T. (1980) Proc. Natl. Acad. Sci. USA, 77, 2542-2545.
12. Ullrich, A., Bell, J. R., Chen, E.Y., Herrera, R., Petruzzelli, L.M., Dull, T.J., Gray, A., Coussens, L., Liao, Y.-C., Tsubokawa, M., Mason, A., Suburg, P.H., Grunfeld, C., Rosen, O.M., and Ramachandran, J. (1985) Nature, 313, 756-761.

Insulin Action and Diabetes,
edited by H. Joseph Goren et al.
Raven Press, New York © 1988.

MONOCLONAL ANTIBODIES AS PROBES OF INSULIN ACTION AND DEGRADATION

Richard A. Roth

Department of Pharmacology, Stanford University
School of Medicine, Stanford, CA 94305

In Dr. Rutter's talk, you heard evidence from molecular biology studies that argues fairly strongly that the tyrosine kinase activity of the insulin receptor is important in mediating insulin's actions (1, 2). Dr. Rosen's group has also performed studies utilizing a molecular approach to demonstrate the role of the receptor kinase in mediating insulin's responses (3). In complementary studies, Dr. David Morgan has used a monoclonal antibody that inhibits the receptor kinase to also argue that the kinase activity of the insulin receptor is important in most, if not all, effects of insulin (4, 5). What I would like to talk about now is how the receptor kinase might be mediating the biological effects of insulin.

In the first slide, I present two different possible mechanisms (Fig. 1). In the first model, the receptor kinase could phosphorylate some exogenous protein (protein x), the phosphorylation of this protein could activate some function of this protein, and this could lead to the various biological effects of insulin. For example, protein x could be either another kinase (serine- or tyrosine-specific) or a phosphatase. According to model 2, the receptor autophosphorylates and this autophosphorylation changes the conformation of the cytoplasmic domain of the β-subunit such that it interacts with protein x to activate its function. Both of these models are consistent with all of the present data on the role of the insulin receptor kinase in insulin action.

However, according to the second model, protein x would not be phosphorylated on a tyrosine residue. This is in contrast to the first model where protein x would be phosphorylated. That the cytoplasmic domain of the insulin receptor is extensively phosphorylated in the intact cells in response to insulin has been well documented (6). Evidence that the conformation of the cytoplasmic domain changes upon phosphorylation comes from studies of the interaction of various antibodies with the receptor (7).

We therefore sought a method to identify protein x which could detect both proteins that were phosphorylated by the insulin receptor as well as those which weren't. The method we have been trying is to use bifunctional cross-linking agents to cross-link proteins in the vicinity of the receptor, such as protein x, with the receptor. The receptor and the cross-linked proteins can then be immunoprecipitated with antibodies to the receptor. If one uses a cleavable bifunctional cross-linking agent, then one can cleave the cross-linker and release the associated proteins.

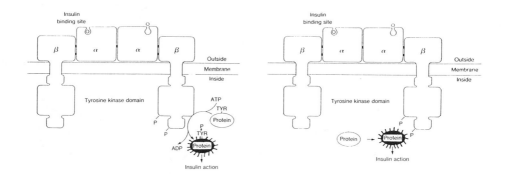

Figure 1. Two models for how the insulin receptor kinase mediates an insulin response. According to both models, the binding of insulin to its receptor activates the intrinsic receptor kinase. In model 1, the receptor kinase then phosphorylates a protein x on a tyrosine residue. Protein x is then activated and mediates the different responses to insulin. In model 2, the receptor kinase autophosphorylates. This autophosphorylation changes the conformation of the cytoplasmic domain of the insulin receptor β subunit such that it can activate protein x. Model 2 differs from model 1 in that only in model 1 is protein x phosphorylated on a tyrosine residue in response to insulin.

———————————————————

Before I show you the data that we have obtained with this approach, I would just like to show you a little bit of data from two other systems which argue that this approach of in vivo cross-linking can be used to identify substrates for various enzymes in the intact cell. You might think, for example, that a bifunctional cross-linking agent will have to cross through the membrane and reach the cytoplasmic side of the receptor to cause this cross-linking, and one might wonder whether one can efficiently do this. Well, in studies with another protein, a metallo-thiol protease which is primarily in the cytosol of cells, we tested this approach. As I am sure all of you know, insulin binds to its receptor and the hormone receptor complexes are internalized (8-14). The internalized vesicles, called endosomes, undergo an acidification process, thereby causing the insulin to dissociate from its receptor. The receptor can then be inactivated or recycled to the plasma membrane. Although extensive studies have been performed on where the internalized insulin goes, it is still not clear what molecules insulin interacts with after internalization.

We therefore decided to try this in vivo cross-linking approach to see if we could cross-link the internalized insulin with proteins it interacts with other than the insulin receptor. One such protein that it might interact with is a specific protease which is in the cytoplasm of cells (15). This protease has been extensively purified and monoclonal antibodies have been produced against it (16, 17). This protease accounts for most of the insulin-degrading activity in cell extracts (15, 17). Also, it can be cross-linked to insulin in vitro (18). To see if we could cross-link the enzyme in vivo, we tried the following approach: Intact living cells were incubated with ^{125}I-insulin for 60 min at 37 degrees, then a bifunctional cross-linking agent (disuccinimidyl suberate) was added to the cells at 4 degrees, and, after an additional 60 min, the cells were lysed and the lysates immunoprecipitated with specific monoclonal antibodies to the insulin-degrading enzyme. The immunoprecipitates were then analyzed by SDS gel electrophoresis to see if the enzyme was cross-linked to ^{125}I-insulin in the intact cell.

When Dr. Joji Hari performed these studies, he found that he could in fact cross-link ^{125}I-insulin to a protein with a Mr = 110,000 by this approach (Fig. 2A, lane 1) (19). This protein is most likely the insulin-degrading enzyme since it has identical molecular weight as this enzyme. In addition, the cross-linked protein was precipitated with specific monoclonal antibodies to this enzyme. The extent of labeling is not very great; however, you wouldn't expect it to be since insulin would be in contact with a protease for only a short period of time before it was degraded. So, to increase the extent of interaction of insulin with the protease and, we hoped, the extent of labeling, we incubated cells with N-ethyl maleimide which inhibits this enzyme and is also a very potent inhibitor of insulin degradation in intact cells (15). What Dr. Hari found was that there was a 500- to 1,000-fold increase in labeling of the insulin-degrading enzyme in the presence of N-ethyl maleimide (Fig. 2A, lane b). In fact, the labeling of this protein is so extensive in these treated cells that it almost equals the labeling of the insulin receptor in these cells under the same conditions (Fig. 2A, lane c). Thus, the cross-linker was able to efficiently cross through the membrane and cause a very extensive cross-linking of insulin with this protease in the cytosol of cells. In addition, a number of other studies further demonstrate that the labeling of the insulin-degrading enzyme in these cross-linking studies requires the normal steps that are involved in the processing of insulin. For example, the labeling of the protease required the prior interaction of insulin with its receptor since it was blocked with either high concentrations of insulin or a monoclonal antibody to the insulin receptor (Fig. 2B). These studies therefore support a role for this protease in the cellular processing of insulin. They also show the utility of this in vivo cross-linking approach.

We have also used this in vivo cross-linking approach to look for substrates for another enzyme. This enzyme interchanges disulfide bonds in vitro and has been proposed to be involved in the formation of disulfide bonds in vivo (20, 21). For example, this enzyme could be involved in catalyzing the formation of the disulfide bonds in the insulin receptor which, as you heard about in Dr. Rutter's talk, has a cysteine-rich region in its extracellular domain. In addition, immunoglobulins have lots of disulfide bonds and there is evidence that this enzyme is

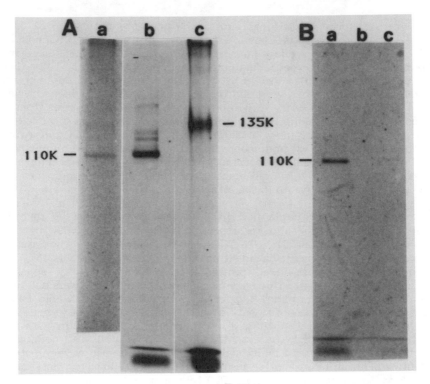

Figure 2. In vivo cross-linking of ^{125}I-insulin to insulin-degrading enzymes. A, Effect of N-ethyl maleimide on the cross-linking. Hep G2 cells were incubated for 1 hour at 37°C in either the presence (b) or absence (a, c) of 0.5 mM N-ethyl maleimide. The cells were then treated with cross-linker at 4°C, lysed and the lysates were precipitated with either antibodies to the degrading enzyme (a, b) or to the insulin receptor (c). B, Cross-linkage of insulin to IDE requires insulin to first bind the insulin receptor. Cells were incubated with ^{125}I-insulin in the presence of either buffer (a), 100 μM insulin (b) or 1 μM of a monoclonal antibody to the hormone binding site of the insulin receptor (c). The cells were then cross-linked and immunoprecipitated with antibodies to the protease. This Fig. was reprinted with permission from Hari et al., Endocrinology 120:829-831, 1987.

---

involved in the formation of disulfide bonds in immunoglobulins (Ig) since it catalyzes this reaction in vitro and the levels of this enzyme increase in lymphocytes actively producing Ig (22). Since this enzyme is in the lumen of the endoplasmic reticulum (ER) (23), the cross-linker would have to go into the cell through the plasma membrane as well as cross through the ER membrane. So it was of interest to see if a cross-linker could get at such a protein, especially since the proteins that the insulin receptor might interact with could be anywhere in the cell.

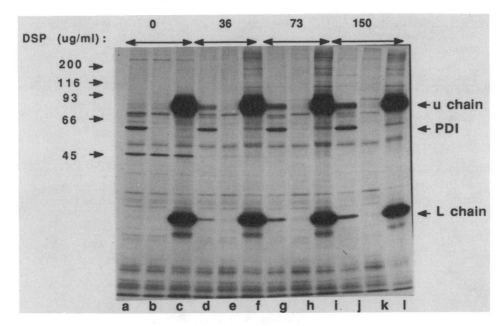

Figure 3. In vivo cross-linking of disulfide interchange enzyme with Igs. Intact lymphocytes were incubated with either no cross-linker (a-c), 35 µg/ml (d-f), 73 µg/ml (g-h) or 150 µg/ml of DSP (j-l), lysed and the lysates immunoprecipitated with either antibodies to the enzyme (a, d, g, j), control Ig (b, e, h, k) or antibodies to mouse Ig (c, f, i, l). Immunoprecipitates were analyzed by SDS gel electrophoresis and autoradiography. This figure has been reprinted with permission from Roth and Pierce, Biochemistry, in press.

And so we tested whether we could also cross-link this enzyme in the intact cell with its potential substrate, immunoglobulins. Again, we found that in the intact cell we could cross-link this enzyme with its proposed substrate. Intact lymphocytes were incubated with different concentrations of a cleavable, bifunctional cross-linker (dithiobis-succinimidylpropionate), lysed, and the lysates were immunoprecipitated with different antibodies (Fig. 3). With increasing amounts of cross-linker there was a dose-dependent co-precipitation of Ig and the enzyme (Fig. 3) (24). In the absence of cross-linker, the two molecules do not co-precipitate.

So these studies argue that this enzyme is involved in synthesis of the disulfide bonds of immunoglobulin. In addition, they argue that the approach of in vivo cross-linking can be used to identify substrates for various enzymes in many different parts of the intact cell. What is surprising is the high efficiency of this cross-linking. For example, in the studies described above, at high cross-linker concentrations, we approached one molecule of immunoglobulin cross-linked per two molecules of the disulfide interchange enzyme (24). This is really a remarkably high efficiency of cross-linking, considering that the cross-linker has to cross two membranes to reach its target.

So, using this approach, we then began looking for a protein x that would interact with the insulin receptor. As I mentioned before, this method should be capable of detecting proteins whether or not they are phosphorylated. We tried a variety of different cross-linkers and different incubation times and conditions, and different labeling procedures. We have been able to identify a single protein of Mr ≈ 250,000 which is cross-linked to the insulin receptor (Fig. 4). We can detect this protein in cells that have been metabolically labeled with [^{35}S]-methionine. We can also detect this protein with antiphosphotyrosine antibodies on a Western. It can be detected only in cells treated with insulin (Fig. 4).

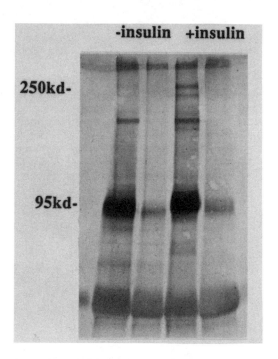

Figure 4. In vivo cross-linking of the insulin receptor with associated proteins. Intact CHO-T cells were incubated with or without insulin, cross-linked, lysed and the lysates were immunoprecipitated with monoclonal anti-receptor antibodies (lanes 1, 3) or control Ig (lanes 2,4). The immunoprecipitates were electrophoresed on SDS gels, transferred to nitrocellulose membranes and probed with antibodies to phosphotyrosine.

We can now isolate this protein since we can cross-link it to the receptor, immunoprecipitate with antibodies to the insulin receptor, and then cleave the cross-linker to release the protein. By utilizing this approach we have isolated some of the protein and can show that it is phosphorylated in vitro by the insulin receptor. We have also shown that the protein is probably a glycoprotein since it binds to a wheat germ agglutinin column. Thus, these studies indicate that a protein of Mr = 250,000 is a substrate for the insulin receptor in vivo and in vitro. In addition, these studies suggest that this protein is in the vicinity of the insulin receptor.

However, as I am sure all of you are aware, this is not the only protein that has been identified that has been shown to be phosphorylated by the insulin receptor (25-27). We have therefore been struggling with the question of how to prove that a particular substrate is important in mediating an insulin response. One approach to testing the role of potential substrates in insulin action is to utilize antibodies to these proteins. If a substrate is important in mediating a response to insulin, antibodies to this substrate might interfere with this response to insulin. However, a limitation to this approach is that one must have antibodies to the potential substrate, preferably antibodies which inhibit the function of the protein. In the case of most substrates for the insulin receptor, these antibodies are not available.

We had previously identified another potential substrate of the insulin receptor by the Sigma-Chemical-Catalogue approach of incubating various proteins with the insulin receptor in vitro and looking to see if they are phosphorylated. The protein we had identified is called ras p21. It is a membrane-bound GTP-binding protein (28), Mr ≈ 21,000, which has been linked through a variety of indirect studies to possibly function in the actions of various growth factors, including epidermal growth factor, platelet-derived growth factor and insulin (29-31). We have found that purified ras p21 could be phosphorylated by the insulin receptor to a limited extent (Fig. 5). When ras p21 is incubated with manganese, ^{32}P-ATP and the insulin receptor, it is phosphorylated, whereas in the absence of receptor it is not. This phosphorylation is most likely on a tyrosine residue since antibodies to phosphotyrosine recognize the phosphorylated ras p21 but not the non-phosphorylated molecule. However, the phosphorylation of ras p21 by the receptor is not very extensive, that is, the stoichiometry of phosphorylation is fairly low. So again we are left with the question of whether this phosphorylation is at all meaningful and if ras p21 is important in mediating the biological responses to insulin.

Well, since ras p21 has been extensively studied, antibodies to this protein have been developed. Frank McCormick and his colleagues had predicted a three-dimensional structure for ras p21 based on analogy with other GTP-binding proteins and had predicted that a particular region which includes residues 15 to 50 would be important in mediating the effects of ras p21 in intact cells (32). Moreover, he and his

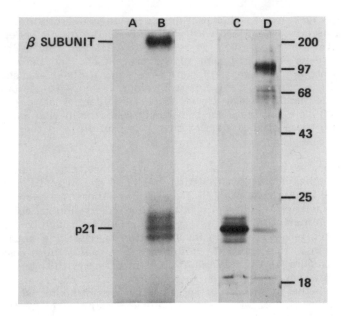

Figure 5. Phosphorylation of ras p21 by purified insulin receptor. Wild-type human N-ras p21 was incubated with either buffer (lane A) or purified insulin receptor (lane b) in the presence of insulin, $MgCl_2$, $MnCl_2$, and $[^{32}P]ATP$. After 1 hour at 24°C, the reaction mixtures were analyzed by SDS gel electrophoresis and autogradiography (lanes A and B). For the experiment shown in lanes C and D, p21 was phosphorylated by purified receptor and analyzed by Western. The nitrocellulose membranes were probed with either monoclonal antibodies to ras p21 (lane C) or polyclonal antibodies to phosphotyrosine (lane D). This Figure has been reprinted from Korn et al., Science 236:840-843.

colleagues have produced a monoclonal antibody to the residues in this region of the ras protein (33). These antibodies would thus be predicted to block ras p21 function in the intact cell. We therefore had an antibody which could be utilized to test the role of ras p21 in insulin action.

The system we chose for these studies was the frog oocyte. Frog oocytes are about 100,000 times the size of mammalian cells and so can be more readily injected with a needle to put the antibody into the cytoplasm of the cells (34). The frog oocytes have been previously shown to have insulin receptors and there are a variety of biological effects of insulin on frog oocytes (35). There are long-term effects of insulin on the oocytes which require six to eight hours to occur, such as the stimulation of germinal vesicle breakdown as seen by formation of a white cap on the frog oocyte. This effect of insulin was previously shown to require the tyrosine kinase activity of the insulin receptor since monoclonal antibodies which inhibit this activity inhibit this response to insulin (4). It has also been shown by Birchmeier et al. that if you inject purified ras p21 into frog oocytes, you can mimic this effect of insulin; that is, ras p21 stimulates germinal vesicle breakdown (36).

These results are consistent with the proposed role of ras p21 in mediating this effect of insulin. To directly test this hypothesis, we examined whether the monoclonal antibodies to ras p21 would block this effect of insulin on the frog oocytes (37). These studies were performed in collaboration with Dr. Laurence Korn and Chris Siebel in the Department of Genetics at Stanford University. The results of these studies are summarized in Fig. 6. The antibodies to ras p21 were found to be very potent inhibitors of insulin's ability to stimulate germinal vesicle breakdown in the frog oocytes. In contrast, control immunoglobulin, at the same concentrations, did not inhibit this effect of insulin.

To test whether the effect of the monoclonal antibody to ras p21 was specific, we utilized progesterone, another hormone that stimulates germinal vesicle breakdown via its own distinct receptor and via a distinct mechanism. The antibodies to ras p21 had no significant effect on progesterone's ability to stimulate germinal vesicle breakdown in the frog oocytes (Fig. 6). These results argue that this effect of the antibody to ras p21 is specific to the insulin response.

To verify that the monoclonal antibody was in fact reacting with a p21-like protein in the frog oocytes, we did an immunoprecipitation and Western from frog oocyte lysates (37). The monoclonal antibody was found to specifically recognize a protein of Mr = 21,000 in the frog oocyte lysate. These results support the hypothesis that these antibodies are reacting with ras p21 in the frog oocytes and the conclusion that ras p21 is somehow involved in mediating the long-term response of the oocytes to insulin.

Clearly, much work remains. It will be important to determine what other responses to insulin are blocked by the monoclonal antibodies to ras p21. Also, it will be necessary to determine whether ras p21 is phosphorylated in the intact cell in response to insulin. If not, it could still be activated by its interaction with the autophosphorylated insulin receptor (as shown in model 2, Fig. 1). Such a mechanism would be similar to that for other GTP-binding proteins. Most interesting is the recent finding of Kamata et al. in which they show that insulin can activate the GTP-binding activity of ras p21 in membrane preparations (38).

So, to summarize the studies you have heard: Insulin interacts primarily with the alpha-subunit of its receptor, somehow transmitting a signal through the membrane which activates the intrinsic kinase activity of the cytoplasmic domain of the beta-subunit. This then initiates the cascade of tyrosine autophosphorylations you heard about from Dr. Kahn and Dr. Avruch. These autophosphorylations of the

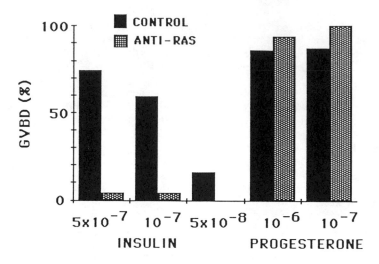

Figure 6. Inhibition of insulin-induced maturation of frog oocytes after microinjection of monoclonal antibodies to ras p21. Frog oocytes were injected with either control Ig (13 μM) or a monoclonal antibody (6B7) to ras p21 (13 μM). These oocytes were then treated with the indicated concentrations of insulin or progesterone, incubated overnight at 19°C, and then analyzed for maturation by the appearance of a white spot in the pigmented animal pole. These data have been adapted from Ref. 37.

---

receptor are somehow important in mediating the biological responses to insulin. It is possible that the receptor kinase phosphorylates another protein, for example, the protein of Mr = 250,000 which we identified in the cross-linking studies. Alternatively, the autophosphorylated receptor may interact with another protein, for example, the ras p21 molecule, and this interaction could activate the GTP-binding activity of this protein. Additional studies are required to further elucidate the role of these proteins as well as others in mediating the various biological responses to insulin.

Thank you.

Acknowledgements

I would like to thank my collaborators, Drs. David Morgan, Joji Hari, Laurence Korn, Chris Siebel, and Frank McCormick, for stimulating discussions and participation in this work; Jacqueline Beaudoin for excellent technical assistance; and Karen Bird for preparation of the manuscript. This work was supported by National Institutes of Health Grant DK34926 and Research Career Development Award DK01393.

REFERENCES

1. Ellis, L., Morgan, D.O., Clauser, E., Roth, R.A., and Rutter, W.J. (1987): Molecular Endocrinology 1:15-24.

2. Ebina, Y., Araki, E., Taira, M., Shimada, F., Mori, M., Craik, C.S., Siddle, K., Pierce, S.B., Roth, R.A., and Rutter, W.J. (1987): Proc. Natl. Acad. Sci. USA 84:704-708.

3. Chou, C.K., Dull, T.J., Russell, D.S., Gherzi, R., Lebwohl, D., Ullrich, A., and Rosen, O.M. J. Biol. Chem. 262:1842-1847.

4. Morgan, D.O., Ho, L., Korn, L.J., and Roth, R.A. (1986): Proc. Natl. Acad. Sci. USA 83:328-332.

5. Morgan, D.O., and Roth, R.A. (1987): Proc. Natl. Acad. Sci. USA 84:41-45.

6. Kahn, C.R. (1985): Ann. Rev. Med. 36:429-451.

7. Morgan, D.O., and Roth, R. A. (1986): Biochemistry 25:1364-1371.

8. Terris, S., and Steiner, D.F. (1975): J. Biol. Chem. 250:8389-8398.

9. Kahn, C.R., and Baird, K. (1978): J. Biol. Chem. 253:4900-4906.

10. Suzuki, K., and Kono, T. (1979): J. Biol. Chem. 254:9786-9794.

11. Marshall, S., and Olefsky, J.M. (1979): J. Biol. Chem. 254:10153-10160.

12. Fan, J.Y., Carpentier, J-L., Gorden, P., Van Obberghen, E., Blackett, N.M., Grunfeld, C., and Orci, L. (1982): Proc. Natl. Acad. Sci. USA 79:7788-7791.

13. Smith, R.M., and Jarett, L. (1983): J. Cell. Physiol. 115:199-207.

14. Khan, M.N., Posner, B.I., Khan, R.J., and Bergeron, J.J.M. (1982): J. Biol. Chem. 257:5969-5976.

15. Duckworth, W.C., and Kitabchi, A.E. (1981): Endo. Rev. 2:210-232.

16. Shii, K., Yokono, K., Baba, S., and Roth, R.A. (1986): Diabetes 35:675-683.

17. Shii, K., and Roth, R.A. (1986): Proc. Natl. Acad. Sci., USA 83:4147-4151.

18. Shii, K., Baba, S., Yokono, K., and Roth, R.A. (1985) J. Biol. Chem. 260:6503-6506.

19. Hari, J., Shii, K., and Roth, R.A. (1987): Endocrinology 120:829-831.

20. Anfinsen, C.B., and Scheraga, H.A. (1975): Adv. Protein Chem. 29:205-300.

21. Edman, J.C., Ellis, L., Blacher, R.W., Roth, R.A., and Rutter, W.J. (1985): Nature 317:267-270.

22. Roth, R.A., and Koshland, M.E. (1981): Biochemistry 20:6594-6599.

23. Freedman, R.B., and Hillson, D.A. (1980): In: The Enzymology of Post-Translational Modifications of Proteins, edited by R.B. Freedman and H.C. Hawkins, pp. 167-212. Academic Press, New York.

24. Roth, R.A., and Pierce, S.B. (1987): Biochemistry (in press).

25. White, M.F., Maron, R., and Kahn, C.R. (1985): Nature 318:183-186.

26. Perrotti, N., Accili, D., Marcus-Samuels, B., Rees-Jones, R.W., and Taylor, S.I. (1987): Proc. Natl. Acad. Sci. USA 84:3137-3140.

27. Kadowaki, T., Koyasu, S., Nishida, E., Tobe, K., Izumi, T., Takaku, F., Sakai, H., Yahara, I., and Kasuga, M. (1987): J. Biol. Chem. 262:7342-7350.

28. Stryer, L., and Bourne, H.R. (1986): Ann. Rev. Cell Biol. 2:391-419.

29. Kamata, T., and Feramisco, J.R. (1984): Nature 110:147-150.

30. Mulcahy, L.S., Smith, M.R., and Stacey, D.W. (1985): Nature 313:241-243.

31. Hagag, N., Halegoua, S., and Viola, M. (1986) Nature 319:680-682.

32. McCormick, F., Clark, B.F.C., la Cour, T.F.M., Kjeldgaard, M., Norskov-Lauritsen, L., and Nyborg, J. (1985): Science 230:78-82.

33. Wong, G., Arnheim, N., Clark, R., McCabe, P., Innis, M., Aldwin, L., Nitecki, D., and McCormick, F. (1986): Cancer Research 46:6029-6033.

34. Gurdon, J.B., and Wickens, M.P. (1983): Methods Enzymol. 101:370-386.

35. Maller, J.L., and Koontz, J.W. (1981): Dev. Biol. 85:309-316.

36. Birchmeier, C., Broek, D., and Wigler, M. (1985): Cell 43:615-621.

37. Korn, L.J., Siebel, C.W., McCormick, F., and Roth, R.A. (1987): Science 236:840-843.

38. Kamata, T., Kathuria, S., and Fujita-Yamaguchi, Y. (1987) Biochem. Biophys. Res. Commun. 144:19-25.

Insulin Action and Diabetes,
edited by H. Joseph Goren et al.
Raven Press, New York © 1988.

THE ROLE OF ENDOSOMAL KINASE ACTIVITY IN INSULIN ACTION

Barry I. Posner, Masood N. Khan and John J.M. Bergeron,

Departments of Medicine and Anatomy, McGill University and the
Royal Victoria Hospital, Montreal, Quebec, H3A 1A1.

INTRODUCTION

From what has been presented at this conference and from much previous work it is evident that two relatively rapid events occur consequent to insulin interaction with its cell surface receptor. These two early events are: (i) activation of the receptor kinase; and (ii) internalization of insulin-receptor complexes into specialized structures constituting the endosomal apparatus. It remains to be seen how these two events relate to very rapid consequences of insulin's interaction with the cell surface, in particular insulin-mediated hyperpolarization of the cell described by Dr. Zierler. Our work has focused, in recent years, on the role that internalization might play in signal transmission to the cell interior.

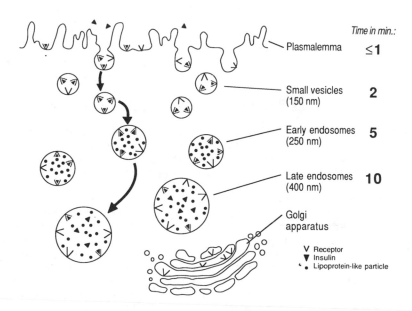

FIGURE 1.   Schematic of insulin-receptor internalization into hepatic endosomes.

Endosomal Apparatus

It is now reasonably well accepted that the insulin-receptor complex formed at the cell surface is rapidly internalized (either with or without apparent microaggregation) into the endosomal compartment of the cell. The endosomal system appears to be heterogeneous (1). Thus, there seems to be a sequence of structures which are involved in the concentrative internalization of ligand. A general outline of the sequence of events involved in internalization is depicted in Figure 1.
This illustrates both the heterogeneity of the system as well as the progressively larger structures in which hormone-receptor complexes accumulate with time. A number of studies have indicated that there is concomitant acidification of the endosomal compartment during the process of internalization (19). Our data have suggested that there is a pH gradient such that early smaller structures are near neutral pH whereas later larger structures develop an acidified interior (8).

Two functions have been attributed to the endosomal apparatus (endosomes): (i) processing of internalized ligands; and (ii) recycling of receptors. In agreement with the study of Pease et al (14) we have shown, in collaboration with Hamel and Duckworth (4), that insulin degradation begins in early endosomes which are near-neutral pH vesicular elements.

The sorting function of endosomes has been well documented in a variety of studies (18). It is clear that the insulin receptor recycles whereas internalized insulin is processed to ultimate degradation, as depicted in Figure 1. Thus, whereas insulin is metabolized rapidly (t $1/2 \approx 10$ minutes) its receptor is metabolized slowly, (t $1/2 \approx 10$ hours) by target cells (11).

Endosomes as Possible Site of Signal Transmission

An interesting additional function for the endosomal system is as a site for signal transmission to the cellular interior. Based on studies of insulin internalization we suggested the possibility that an activated form of receptor may carry out specific functions inside the cell (15).

In recent years both biochemical and genetic studies have led to the elucidation of the structure of the insulin receptor and the demonstration that the β-subunit contains a tyrosine kinase activity on its cytoplasmic domain (2,20). Rosen and her collaborators showed that insulin, on binding to the α-subunit of the receptor, augmented the kinase activity on the β-subunit (16). Furthermore it was demonstrated that this augmented activity persisted after the subsequent removal of insulin and thus reflected an activated state of the receptor kinase (9,10,22). The activated state was shown to be dependent upon autophosphorylation of the receptor on its β-subunit (7). A mutagenized receptor in which tyrosine residues 1162 and 1163 on the β-subunit of the receptor were replaced by phenylalanine, bound insulin adequately but could not be significantly activated as a consequence and mediated a considerably reduced biological response (13). Replacement of lysine 1030 by alanine not only inactivated the receptor kinase completely but abolished the ability of the insulin receptor to mediate insulin action (17). In other studies antibodies to the kinase domain, when concentrated intracellularly, markedly inhibited insulin action (12). Finally, insulin mimickers such as vanadate, H2O2 and pervanadate both activate the receptor kinase and promote insulin action (5,6). This latter phenomenon is illustrated in Fig 2.

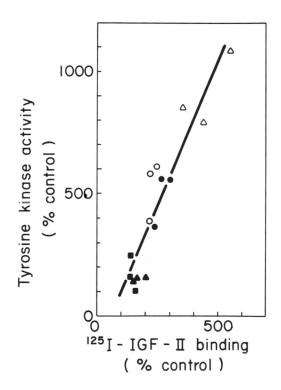

FIGURE 2. Insulin and insulin-mimickers augment both insulin receptor tyrosine kinase activity and fat cell surface IGF receptors. For experimental details consult reference (16) from which this figure has been obtained. Rat adipocytes were incubated with insulin (10 ng/ml) (●), vanadate (1 mM) (▲), H_2O_2 (1 mM) (■), insulin (10 ng/ml) + H_2O_2 (1 mM) (o) or vanadate (1 mM) + H_2O_2 (1 mM) (Δ). Linear correlation was r=0.927 (n=15) at p < 0.001.

Here we have studied the efficacy of insulin and various insulin mimickers to promote translocation of IGF receptor from intracellular sites to the cell surface. In examining this well-documented action of insulin (21) we have correlated it with the change in kinase activity promoted by insulin and the insulin mimickers (6). The strong correlation between biological response and activation of kinase is evident and lends further support to the key role for kinase in realizing insulin action.

Our working hypothesis has been that the activated kinase is internalized. As depicted in Fig. 3 the internalization process is associated with a continuing cytoplasmic orientation of the kinase domain of the insulin receptor. Furthermore the key role for receptor internalization in being able to interact with topographically discrete substrates is illustrated. The binding site is enclosed within endosomes and sequestered from the cytosolic environment. Thus freshly isolated intact endosomes are unable to bind insulin and must be permeabilized, either by freeze-thawing or a low concentration of Triton X-100, to permit <u>in vitro</u> hormone-receptor interaction. The studies to be

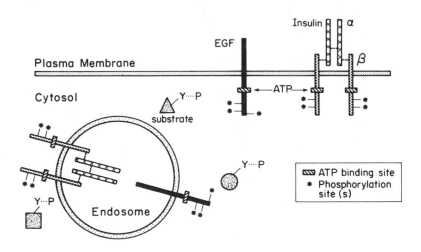

FIGURE 3. Orientation of receptor kinases in plasma membrane (PM) and endosome. Note that internalization leads to sequestration of ligand binding domains and continuous cytosolic orientation of receptor kinase domains. The likely aggregation during internalization of EGF receptors in particular is not depicted for simplicity.

described below have all been done with freshly isolated subcellular fractions that consist of intact endosomes, free of significant plasma membrane contamination, or a purified plasma membrane preparation (9).

The basic experimental paradigm has involved the administration of insulin to male rats by intrajugular injection. In our initial studies we employed a dose of 150 ug/100 gm bdy. wt. Endosomes were prepared 15 minutes post-injection, were solubilized, and the insulin receptor was partially purified by wheat germ agglutinin (WGA)-Sepharose chromatography. The capacity of insulin receptors from both uninjected and insulin-treated animals to carry out autophosphorylation after partial purification was assessed by incubations with ^{32}P-ATP (9). On terminating the phosphorylation reaction the receptor was immunoprecipitated and resolved by gel electrophoresis. Autoradiograms of these gels illustrated considerably augmented activity of receptors from insulin-treated animals. These observations are summarized in Table 1 where it is also shown that the increased activity persisted in the presence of excess antibody to insulin which completely abolished the effect of exogenously administered insulin to augment in vitro insulin receptor kinase activity. This latter observation confirms that little internalized insulin remained associated with endosomal receptors following solubilization and WGA chromatographic purification. Thus, the augmented activity was not an artifact of insulin "carried through" the purification but reflected a genuine activation of the receptor. The augmented activity following insulin injection was shown to be dose dependent and evident when exogenous substrate phosphorylation was studied as well. Furthermore, the specificity of in vivo activation was established since parallel injections of human growth hormone,

TABLE 1. Insulin-stimulated autophosphorylation in hepatic endosomes: effect of antiserum to insulin on kinase activity

Insulin Administered		Antiserum	
In vivo	In vitro	-	+
-	-	2	4
-	+	100	7
+	-	62	78

Endosomes were prepared 15 min. after insulin or saline injection. Partially purified receptors were subjected to autophosphorylation in the presence and absence of $10^{-7}M$ insulin plus or minus insulin antiserum. Kinase activity (autophosphorylation) is expressed as a percent of the maximum seen with an excess (100 nM) of in vitro insulin. For details of autophosphorylation determination consult reference 9 from which these data were adapted.

glucagon or EGF did not affect basal autophosphorylation activity of the insulin receptor.

In our most recent studies we have examined the time course of receptor kinase activation in plasma membrane (cell surface) and endosomes (internalized receptor). In these studies we have injected 1.5 ug of insulin/100 gm bdy. wt., a dose resulting in approximately 40% occupancy of hepatocyte cell surface receptors (15). At timed intervals after this injection (0.5, 1, 5, 10 and 20 minutes) animals were sacrificed and both plasma membrane and endosomal fractions were isolated from liver. The isolated membrane fractions were incubated directly in a phosphorylation assay containing ^{32}P-ATP. The ^{32}P-labeled membranes were solubilized, the insulin receptor immunoprecipitated, and the immunoprecipitate analysed by gel electrophoresis followed by radioautography and quantitative densitometry. In parallel with estimates of phosphorylation by intact membrane fractions, experiments were done evaluating kinase activity of solubilized partially purified (WGA-affinity chromatography) receptor obtained from the membranes. These partially purified receptors were analysed both for autophosphorylation and for the ability to phosphorylate a synthetic substrate (polyGlu:Tyr). Time course studies indicated that kinase activity was maximal in plasma membrane fractions 30 seconds after insulin injection. At this time it was possible to observe a dose-dependent stimulation of kinase activity by insulin. In endosomes the maximal activity was observed at 2-5 minutes following insulin injection. Here too the extent of activation was dose-dependent and in both plasma membrane and endosomes kinase activation could be seen at doses as low as 50 ng/100 gm bdy. wt. The time course of activation in both plasma membrane and endosomes was the same whether intact membranes were studied or whether the analysis was performed on partially purified receptors. In latter preparations the relative activities of either autophosphorylation or exogenous substrate phosphorylation were very similar. Thus these studies indicate a true in vivo activation of the receptor kinase at doses of insulin in the physiologic range. Phosphatase treatment of these cell fractions abolished the activated state of the receptor indicating the reversibility of activation and the importance of receptor phosphorylation in achieving the activated state in vivo. In Figure 4 we depict a model of phosphorylation dependent receptor activation, following insulin binding, in which the receptor becomes activated at the cell surface followed by its internalization or may undergo activation during the course of internalization. This process would not preclude liberation of second messengers during the course of receptor activation and internalization.

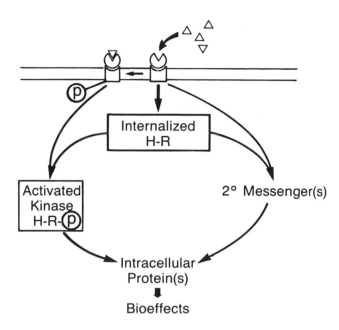

FIGURE 4.   Phosphorylation-dependent activation of the insulin receptor kinase.   Activation may occur on the cell surface and/or following internalization.

Further studies have examined the relationship between the maximal level of kinase activity in the plasma membrane versus the maximal level in the endosome.   Thus autophosphorylation activity in both intact membranes and partially purified receptors was determined for plasma membrane 30 seconds after insulin   injection   and   for   endosomes   at   5   minutes post-injection.   On average, we observed a 6-7 fold greater activation of autophosphorylation in the endosomal fraction, relative to the plasma membrane fraction.   These data point to the endosome as being a site of special significance or interest in respect to kinase activity.   In further studies we compared maximal   activities   in   respect   to   exogenous   substrate phosphorylation.   Kinetic analysis indicate that for plasma membranes activation was associated with an increase in Vmax and an increase in Km.   In contradistinction activation of endosomal receptors produced an increase in Vmax with an appreciable decrease in Km.   To present these data in a compact way we depict them in Table 2 in respect to Vmax/Km.   This ratio should be an index of the degree of kinase activation and its use is justified on the basis that the initial velocity of an enzyme

TABLE 2.　Effect of in vivo insulin on receptor kinase activity

	Vmax/Km	
Fold over	PM	ENs
Control	2.5 ± 0.4	20.2 ± 6.1

Insulin receptors were partially purified from endosomes (ENs) at 5 min. and from plasma membrane (PM) at 30 sec after i.v. insulin (1.5 ug/100 g. bdy. wt.) or saline. Kinetic parameters were determined for both control (saline) and activated (+ insulin) receptors in an exogenous substrate (poly Glu:Tyr) assay described in reference 6. Vmax/Km was determined for control and activated receptors from PM and ENs. The fold increase in Vmax/Km in activated versus control receptors is depicted in the Table. The increase in Vmax/Km for ENs is almost 10 times that seen in PM (p < 0.02, N=3).

reaction is proportional to V max and inversely proportional to Km at very low substrate concentrations. The data indicate that the ratio of Vmax/Km is increased consequent to insulin injection but that this increase is far greater for endosomal receptors than for plasma membrane receptors. These results can be interpreted as being compatible with the data on autophosphorylation.

The possibility of activation occuring in relationship to the internalization process is intriguing. How might such activation occur? Two models, which are not mutually exclusive, are: (i) an activation model; and (ii) a concentration model (Fig.5). In the first instance insulin binds to the α -subunit and triggers the kinase, thereby beginning receptor activation. However, the initial activation state is hypothesized to be minimal. In this model internalization is coupled to some chemical alteration of the receptor which activates it further and produces an augmented specific activity of the receptor in endosomes. The second model postulates that there is a heterogeneous population of cell surface insulin receptors in terms of their ability to undergo ligand-dependent activation. On binding insulin only receptors which can be fully activated are the ones which concentrate intracellularly. This postulate is supported by recent data on a mutagenized insulin receptor, in which lysine 1030 was replaced by alanine, which could neither be activated nor internalized (17). This model does not suggest that activated receptors are the only ones to be internalized but requires that they are the ones which end up being selectively concentrated in endosomes. Both models postulate a role for the endosome and its highly activated kinase in signal transmission. Nonetheless, in terms of the overall action of insulin, the model must consider some activity of the kinase at the cell surface. Thus, the observations of

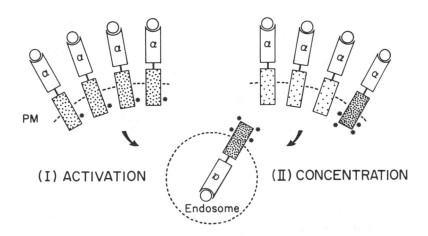

FIGURE 5. Endosomal accumulation of activated insulin receptor kinase. Two mutually nonexclusive mechanisms of activation and concentration are depicted.

Morrison and Pessin suggesting that insulin can stimulate receptor kinase activity without autophosphorylation of the receptor (13) would imply a role for the receptor in its minimally activated state.

In summary, it would appear that the two early events which occur after insulin binding to its receptor, namely the activation of the kinase and its internalization appear to be intimately related. At least in the hepatocyte in vivo the data which we have obtained strongly suggest that a highly activated form of the kinase is concentrated in endosomes. This observation is consistent with an important role for the endosome in mediating the biological effect of insulin.

ACKNOWLEDGEMENTS

This work has been supported by grants from the U.S. Public Health Service and the Medical Research Council of Canada.

REFERENCES

1. Bergeron, J.J.M., Cruz, J., Khan, M.N., and Posner, B.I. (1985): Annual Rev. Physiol. 3:383-403.
2. Ebina, Y., Ellis, L., Jarnagin, K., Edery, M., Graf, L., Clauser, E., Ou, J.-H., Maslarz, F., Kan, Y.W., Goldfine, I.D., Roth, R.A., and Rutter, W.J. (1985): Cell 40:747-758.
3. Ellis, L., Clauser, E., Morgan, D.O., Edery, M., Roth, R.A., and Rutter, W.J. (1986): Cell 45:721-732.
4. Hamel, F.G., Posner, B.I., Bergeron, J.J.M., Frank, B.H., and Duckworth, W.C. (manuscript submitted for publication).
5. Kadota, S., Fantus, I.G., Deragon, G., Guyda, H.J., Hersh, B., and Posner, B.I. (1987): Biochem. Biophys. Res. Commun. 147:259-266.
6. Kadota, S., Fantus, I.G., Deragon, G., Guyda, H.J., and Posner, B.I. (1987): J. Biol. Chem. 262:8252-8256.
7. Khan, M.N., Baquiran, G., Brule, C., Vanderwele, M., Foster, B., Bergeron, J.J.M., and Posner, B.I. (manuscript submitted for publication).
8. Khan, M.N., Savoie, S., Bergeron, J.J.M., and Posner, B.I. (1985): Diabetes 34:1025-1030.
9. Khan, M.N., Savoie, S., Bergeron, J.J.M., and Posner, B.I. (1986): J. Biol. Chem. 261:8462-8472.
10. Klein, H.H., Friedenberg, G.R., Kladde, M., and Olefsky, J.M. (1986): J. Biol. Chem. 261:4691-4697.
11. Krupp, M., and Lane, M.D. (1981): J. Biol. Chem. 256:1689-1694.
12. Morgan, D.D., and Roth, R.A. (1987): Proc. Natl. Acad. Sci. U.S.A. 84:41-45.
13. Morrison, B.D., and Pessin, J.E. (1987): J. Biol. Chem. 262:2861-1868.
14. Pease, R.J., Smith, G.D., and Peters, T.J. (1985): Biochem. J. 228:137-146.
15. Posner, B.I., Patel, B., Verma, A.K., and Bergeron, J.J.M. (1980): J. Biol. Chem. 255:735-741.
16. Rosen, O.M., Herrera, R., Olowe, Y., Petruzzelli, L.M. and Cobb, M.H. (1983): Proc. Natl. Acad. Sci. U.S.A. 80:3232-3240.
17. Russell, D.S., Gherzi, R., Johnson, E.L., Chou, C.-K, and Rosen, O.M. (1987): J. Biol. Chem. 262:11833-11840.
18. Stahl, P., and Schwartz, A.L. (1986): J. Clin. Invest. 77:657-662.
19. Tycko, B., and Maxfield, F.R. (1982): 28:643-651.
20. Ullrich, A., Bell, J.R., Chen, E.Y., Herrera, R., Petruzzelli, L.M., Dull, T.J., Gray, A., Coussens, L., Liao, Y.-C., Tsubokawa, M., Mason, A., Seeburg, P.H., Grunfeld, C., Rosen, O.M., and Ramachandran, J. (1985): Nature 313:756-761.
21. Wardzala, L.J., Simpson, I.A., Rechler, M.M., and Cushman, S.W. (1984): J. Biol. Chem. 259:8378-8383.
22. Yu, K.-T, and Czech, M.P. (1986): J. Biol. Chem. 261:4715-4722.

Insulin Action and Diabetes,
edited by H. Joseph Goren et al.
Raven Press, New York © 1988.

SUBCELLULAR DISTRIBUTION OF INSULIN RECEPTOR

TYROSINE KINASE ACTIVITY IN RAT ADIPOSE CELLS

T.M. Weber, S. DiPaolo, H.G. Joost, S.W. Cushman, and I.A. Simpson

Experimental Diabetes, Metabolism and Nutrition Section, MCNEB/NIDDK,
National Institutes of Health, Bethesda, MD 20892, USA.

The phosphorylation state and tyrosine kinase activity of insulin receptors were analyzed after exposure of intact cells to insulin. Insulin induced a 6 to 7-fold phosphorylation of cell-surface insulin receptors. Phosphorylation was maintained upon receptor internalization into high- and low-density microsomes. Likewise, the tyrosine kinase activity of plasma membrane and intracellular receptors was enhanced by insulin, with similar half maximal stimulating concentrations for all three fractions. However, the maximal kinase activity was approximately 50% lower in low-density compared to high-density microsomes and plasma membranes. Thus, insulin receptors retain their kinase activity upon internalization, suggesting that the receptor kinase might mediate insulin's effects while inside the cell. However, if the internalized receptor kinase mediates insulin's effect on glucose transport, only a portion of its maximal kinase activity (<20%) appears to be necessary for full transport stimulation. Further, the difference in kinase activity among subfractions suggests that the receptor kinase in low-density microsomes may be in the process of deactivation.

INTRODUCTION

Insulin triggers a rapid activation of the insulin receptor tyrosine kinase in isolated rat adipocytes. Occupied, activated receptors are internalized and can be identified in subcellular membrane fractions. The present study was performed to investigate whether these internalized insulin receptors retain their phosphorylation state and tyrosine kinase activity, and thus might mediate some of insulin's effects through an intracellular pathway. Specifically, the insulin concentration dependence of receptor kinase activation in both plasma membranes and intracellular membrane fractions was compared with insulin's ability to stimulate glucose transport activity.

151

METHODS

Isolated adipocytes were incubated with varying concentrations of insulin for 30 min and homogenized in the presence of phosphatase inhibitors to preserve their phosphorylation state. Subcellular fractionation (5,7) yielded plasma membranes (PM), and two receptor containing intracellular pools, high-density microsomes (HDM) and low-density microsomes (LDM). Glucose transport activity was measured in plasma membrane vesicles by a rapid filtration assay (7). Insulin receptor binding was determined in wheat germ eluates and tyrosine kinase activity was measured by [^{32}P]phosphate incorporation into the synthetic heteropolymeric substrate, (4:1) Glu:Tyr (8).

In addition, receptor autophosphorylation in intact adipose cells was studied by prelabeling isolated cells with [^{32}P]phosphate prior to adding a maximally stimulating concentration of insulin. Insulin receptors from each of the membrane fractions were then immunoprecipitated with an anti-receptor antiserum (B-2). The phosphorylated β-subunit was visualized by autoradiography of the immunoprecipitates following SDS-PAGE.

RESULTS

To preserve the phosphorylation state of insulin receptors recovered in adipocyte subfractions, isolated cells were homogenized and fractionated in the presence of a phosphatase inhibitor cocktail. Figure 1 demonstrates the insulin-induced loss of insulin receptors from PM, and their subsequent incorporation into high- and low-density microsomes. This redistribution was similar to receptor internalization observed when cells were fractionated in the absence of phosphatase inhibitors (6). Thus, the

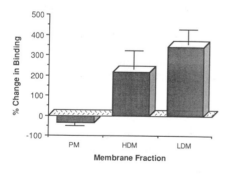

FIG. 1. Redistribution of insulin receptors in rat adipocytes in response to a maximally stimulating concentration of insulin. Cell suspensions (1.2 x 10^6 cells/ml) were incubated for 30 min with 0 or 81 nM insulin. The cells were then washed with homogenization buffer (20 mM Tris, 1 mM EDTA, 255 mM sucrose, 10 mM sodium fluoride, 10 mM sodium pyrophosphate and 0.2 mM sodium vanadate, pH 7.4), homogenized and fractionated by differential centrifugation into PM, HDM, and LDM. Insulin receptors were partially purified from Triton X-100 solubilized membrane fractions adsorbed to wheat germ agarose. Eluates of each of the membrane fractions were then incubated with tracer ^{125}I-insulin ± 17.0 μM insulin at 4°C overnight. Bound and free insulin were separated by polyethylene glycol precipitation of insulin:receptor complexes, and radioactivity was counted. Data shown are normalized for protein concentration and for receptor concentration in the basal state, and represent the means ± S.E. of 3 experiments.

presence of phosphatase inhibitors in this study affected neither membrane fractionation nor receptor recovery in adipocyte subfractions. Furthermore, in the presence of phosphatase inhibitors, the phosphorylation state of several insulin-sensitive proteins, as well as proteins not specifically modulated by insulin was maintained (Fig. 2).

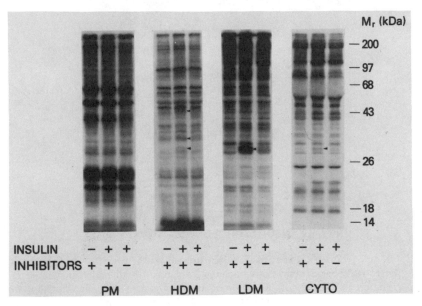

FIG. 2. Effect of insulin and phosphatase inhibitors on [^{32}P]phosphate incorporation into subfractions of rat adipocytes. Cells were labeled with sodium [^{32}P]phosphate (0.1 mM, 0.1 mCi/ml) for 80 min, then incubated for an additional 30 min ± 10 nM insulin. Crude membrane fractions were prepared from cells prelabeled as described and incubated with and without insulin (10 nM). Phosphatase inhibitors were included in the homogenization buffer (as indicated in the legend of Fig. 1). *Arrows* indicate insulin-stimulated phosphate incorporation sensitive to the presence of phosphatase inhibitors.

Under these conditions, insulin stimulated a 6 to 7-fold phosphorylation of cell surface insulin receptors (Fig. 3). Receptors which were internalized into HDM and LDM as a result of insulin incubation were also highly phosphorylated. However, the fold-response could not accurately be measured due to low basal signals. Insulin receptors from each of the membrane fractions also expressed tyrosine kinase activity stimulated by insulin treatment of the intact cell (Fig. 4). All three fractions exhibited similar dose dependence (EC$_{50}$'s: PM, 4.1 ± 0.34; HDM, 2.4 ± 0.5; LDM,

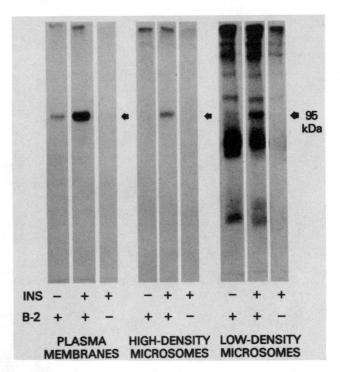

FIG. 3.   Insulin   receptor   autophosphorylation   in   intact   cells.
[^{32}P]phosphate-labeled membrane fractions from basal and insulin-stimulated cells
were prepared as described.   Equal amounts of protein (within each fraction) were
solubilized   and   incubated   overnight   with   B-2   *(+)*,   a   human   anti-insulin   receptor
antiserum, or human control serum *(-)*, at dilutions of 1:300.   The phosphorylated
β-subunit (95 kDa) was visualized by autoradiography of the immunoprecipitates
following SDS-PAGE on 7% reducing gels.   The data are representative of 3
experiments.

2.77 ± 0.69 nM, means ± S.E.), although the activity in LDM did not attain
the same maximum as that observed in PM and HDM (maximal activity per
LDM receptor = 56 ± 5.4% of that in PM).

A comparison of insulin receptor kinase activation and plasma membrane
glucose transport stimulation is shown in Fig. 5.   Transport *(filled circles)*
was maximally stimulated at a concentration of insulin (1.0 nM) which
resulted in <20% of the maximal kinase activity *(open circles)*.   Transport
stimulation has been reported to exhibit an EC_{50} of 0.1 nM (4) in intact
adipose cells, compared to the greater than 10-fold higher EC_{50}'s for kinase
activation observed in PM, or LDM (the intracellular compartment from
which glucose transporters are recruited in response to insulin, 1).

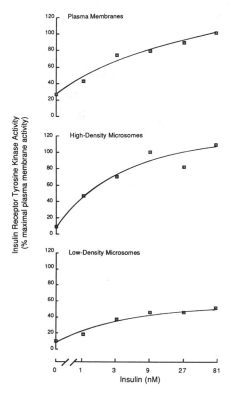

FIG. 4. Insulin receptor tyrosine kinase activity in subcellular fractions isolated from rat adipose cells pretreated with insulin. Isolated adipose cells were incubated (with the indicated concentrations of insulin) as described in the legend of Fig. 1, and membrane fractions were prepared. Insulin receptors were partially purified by adsorption to wheat germ agglutinin and were incubated for 10 min at room temperature with 4 μM [^{32}P]ATP (1 μCi/sample) and the synthetic substrate poly-Glu/Tyr (4:1 polymer, 2.2 mg/ml). The samples were adsorbed onto filter papers, washed in 10% TCA/10 mM sodium pyrophosphate, dried and counted. Data shown are normalized for insulin receptor number and then compared to the maximal activity observed in plasma membrane derived receptors. The figure shows a representative experiment which was repeated 3 times.

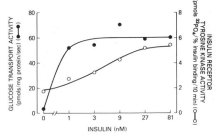

FIG. 5. Comparison of insulin receptor kinase activation with glucose transport stimulation in plasma membranes from adipocytes pretreated with insulin. Glucose transport activity in plasma membrane vesicles prepared from insulin-stimulated cells *(filled circles)* was assayed by a previously described rapid filtration equilibrium exchange procedure (7). Tyrosine kinase activity *(open circles)* was determined in partially purified insulin receptor derived from plasma membranes, as described above. The data are from one representative experiment which was repeated 3 times.

CONCLUSIONS

In the insulin-stimulated rat adipocyte, intracellular insulin receptors exhibit both an enhanced phosphorylation state and a stimulated tyrosine kinase activity, and therefore may be capable of mediating insulin's effects through an intracellular pathway. However, the extent of receptor kinase stimulation in LDM appears to be considerably lower than that in HDM and PM, suggesting a deactivation in the LDM. Furthermore, the insulin concentration dependencies of kinase activation in LDM and of glucose transport stimulation in PM differ by more than a factor of 10. Therefore, if internalized receptor kinase activity is responsible for initiation of the glucose transporter translocation process, the kinase signal must be amplified since the transporter itself is not phosphorylated in response to insulin (2,3).

REFERENCES

1. Cushman, S.W., and Wardzala, L.J. (1980): *J. Biol. Chem.,* 255:4758-4762.
2. Gibbs, E.M., Allard, W.J., and Lienhard, G.E. (1986): *J. Biol. Chem.,* 261:16597-16603.
3. Joost, H.G., Weber, T.M., Cushman, S.W., and Simpson, I.A. (1987): *J. Biol. Chem.,* 262:11261-11267.
4. Karnieli, E., Zarnowski, M.J., Hissin, P.J., Simpson, I.A., Salans, L.B., and Cushman, S.W. (1981): *J. Biol. Chem.,* 256:4772-4777.
5. Simpson, I.A., Yver, D.R., Hissin, P.J., Wardzala, L.J., Karnielli, E., Salans, L.B., Cushman, S.W. (1983): *Biochim. Biophys. Acta* 763: 393-407.
6. Sonne, O., and Simpson, I.A. (1984): *Biochim. Biophys. Acta* 804:404-413.
7. Weber, T.M., Joost, H.G., Simpson, I.A., and Cushman, S.W. (1988): In: *Receptor Biochemistry and Methodology,* edited by C.R. Kahn and L.C. Harrison, (in press). Alan R. Liss, New York.
8. Zick, Y., Rees-Jones, R.W., Taylor, S.I., Gordon, P., and Roth, J. (1984): *J. Biol. Chem.,* 259:4396-4400.

Insulin Action and Diabetes,
edited by H. Joseph Goren et al.
Raven Press, New York © 1988.

PHOSPHORYLATION STATE AND INTRINSIC ACTIVITY

OF GLUCOSE TRANSPORTERS IN PLASMA MEMBRANES

FROM INSULIN-, ISOPROTERENOL-, AND PHORBOL

ESTER-TREATED RAT ADIPOSE CELLS

H. G. Joost, T. M. Weber, I. A. Simpson, and S. W. Cushman

Experimental Diabetes, Metabolism, and Nutrition Section, MCNEB/NIDDK,
National Institutes of Health, Bethesda, MD 20892, USA.

Neither insulin nor isoproterenol induced any detectable phosphate incorporation into immunoprecipitated glucose transporter from adipose cells equilibrated with $[^{32}P]$phosphate in spite of marked changes in plasma membrane glucose transport activity. In contrast, phorbol ester treatment of insulin-stimulated cells gave rise to significant phosphorylation of plasma membrane transporters. However, phorbol ester failed to alter glucose transporter activity or subcellular distribution. Thus, the phosphorylation state of the glucose transporter is not involved in signaling transporter translocation or mediating changes in transporter intrinsic activity.

INTRODUCTION

Hormonal regulation of glucose transport activity in the adipose cell is achieved by at least two different mechanisms. Insulin stimulates the translocation of glucose transporters from an intracellular pool to the plasma membrane (1). In contrast, catecholamines reduce (and adenosine increases) the intrinsic activity of plasma membrane glucose transporters without changing their concentration, as assessed by the cytochalasin B binding assay (4). The molecular basis of both mechanisms is as yet unknown. In the present study, we investigated the role of phosphorylation of the glucose transporter in regulating transporter translocation and/or intrinsic activity. In addition, the effect of activation of protein kinase C on glucose transport activity and transporter translocation has been studied.

METHODS

Adipose cells were isolated according to the method of Rodbell (6) with modifications as described (8). After preincubation of cells as indicated, membrane fractions were prepared by differential centrifugation (7,8) of the cell homogenate. Stereospecific glucose transport activity in cells and plasma membranes was determined with 3-0-methylglucose (8) or D-glucose (4,8), respectively. Glucose transporter concentrations were determined by the cytochalasin B binding assay (8) and by immunoblotting with antiserum raised against the human erythrocyte glucose transporter (9). Immunoprecipitation of glucose transporter was carried out as described with the α-GT antiserum (3, courtesy of Dr. H. C. Haspel).

RESULTS

In plasma membranes isolated from cells treated with insulin, the initial D-glucose transport rate was stimulated 15-fold as compared to that in membranes from basal cells (Fig. 1, *right panel*). Isoproterenol treatment

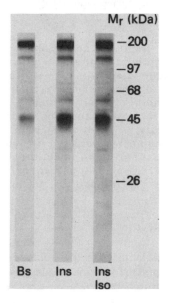

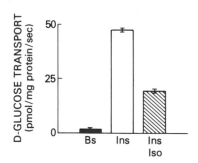

FIG. 1. Immunoblot and transport activity of glucose transporters in plasma membranes from adipose cells treated with insulin and isoproterenol (reproduced from 5). Cells were incubated with insulin (10 nM) for 25 min, and subsequently for 15 min with isoproterenol (0.5 µM) and adenosine deaminase (2.5 µg / ml). Fast shaking speeds and buffers containing 5% albumin were employed in order to prevent accumulation of fatty acids (4). KCN, which is necessary to preserve the inhibitory effect of isoproterenol in the plasma membrane preparation, was added to a final concentration of 2 mM, and the cells were homogenized and fractionated by differential centrifugation. *Left panel,* immunoreactivity of the glucose transporter after Western blotting of membrane fractions. ^{125}I-protein A counts incorporated into the 45 kDa band were 358 (basal), 1201 (insulin) and 1198 cpm (insulin plus isoproterenol). The *right panel* shows the initial D-glucose uptake rate in plasma membrane vesicles from the same, representative membrane preparation as means ± S.E. of triplicate samples. *Bs*, basal; *Ins*, insulin; *Iso*, isoproterenol.

of insulin-stimulated cells (in the presence of adenosine deaminase) reduced the transport activity by approximately 55%. The concentration of glucose transporters as assessed by immunoblotting (*left panel*, Fig. 1) was increased in response to insulin, accounting for the stimulation of plasma membrane glucose transport, but was not altered by isoproterenol.

In cells equilibrated with $[^{32}P]$ phosphate, insulin stimulated the phosphorylation of a 113 kDa low-density microsomal protein, and of at least three cytosolic proteins (45, 43, and 20 kDa, Fig. 2). Isoproterenol stimulated the phosphorylation of a 19 kDa and a 64 kDa protein in plasma membranes and low-density microsomes, respectively. Further, in parallel to its inhibitory effect on glucose transport, the catecholamine counteracted the insulin-stimulated phosphorylation of the cytosolic proteins. However,

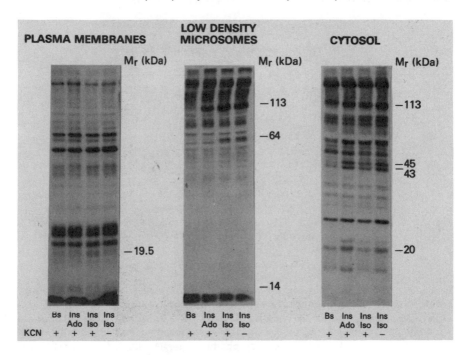

FIG. 2. **Phosphorylation of adipose cells proteins in response to insulin and isoproterenol (reproduced from 5).** Isolated adipose cells were incubated in the presence of $[^{32}P]$sodium phosphate (0.1 mCi/ml, total phosphate concentration 0.1 mM) for 80 min, and insulin ± isoproterenol were added according to the protocol outlined in the legend of Fig. 1. Prior to homogenization, cells were treated with 2 mM KCN where indicated. Membrane fractions were isolated as described, and were separated on SDS-PAGE. As a control for the effects of the agents on glucose transport under the conditions of prelabeling, transport was assayed in plasma membranes which had been stored in liquid nitrogen for at least 4 months (8 ^{32}P half-lives). The transport activity was 5.0 ± 1.2 pmol/mg protein/sec in basal membranes, 37.4 ± 10.8 in membranes from insulin treated cells, and 20.3 ± 3.6 after isoproterenol treatment (means ± S.E.).

neither insulin nor isoproterenol gave rise to any detectable [^{32}P]phosphate incorporation into the glucose transporter from plasma membranes or low-density microsomes (Fig. 3).

Addition of phorbol 12-myristate 13-acetate (PMA) to insulin-stimulated cells increased the [^{32}P]phosphate content of the plasma membrane glucose transporter (Fig. 3). No detectable phosphate incorporation into glucose transporters from low-density microsomes was observed in response to phorbol ester (Fig. 3, *right panel).* In control experiments performed with unlabeled cells according to the protocol which gave rise to phosphorylation of transporters (i.e. preincubation with insulin, subsequent treatment with phorbol ester), phorbol ester failed to alter either intrinsic activity or subcellular distribution of glucose transporters (Fig. 4).

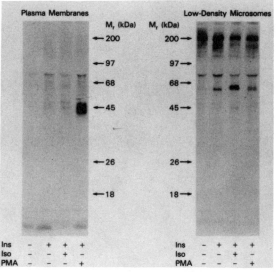

FIG. 3.   Phosphorylation of glucose transporter in adipose cells treated with insulin, isoproterenol, or phorbol ester. Isolated adipose cells were prelabeled with [^{32}P]phosphate (0.1 mCi/ml, total phosphate concentration 0.1mM) for 80 min. Cells were exposed to insulin (10 nM) for 25 min, and thereafter to isoproterenol or phorbol ester (1 μM) for another 15 min. After isolation of plasma membranes *(left panel)* and low-density microsomes *(right panel)*, fractions were solubilized (3) and incubated with antiserum for 16 h, and immunocomplexes were separated with protein A sepharose. Immunoprecipitates were separated on SDS-PAGE. The figure shows autoradiographs of a representative experimental series which was performed 5 times (insulin, isoproterenol) and 3 times (phorbol ester), with similar results. Control immunoprecipitates (not shown) were performed with normal rabbit serum and failed to show any phosphate incorporation in the 45 kDa region. Aliquots of the immunoprecipitates from each experiment were run separately on SDS-PAGE and were immunoblotted with a second antiserum against the glucose transporter in order to control for the transporter concentration in the immunoprecipitates. These controls yielded results comparable with those from experiments in unlabeled cells (Fig. 1 & 4).

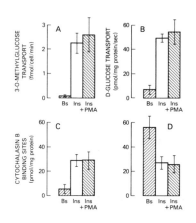

FIG. 4. Effect of PMA on glucose transport activity in adipose cells and plasma membranes, and on subcellular transporter distribution (reproduced from 5). Isolated adipose cells were incubated with insulin where indicated, for 25 min, and thereafter with PMA (1μM), for another 15 min. Glucose transport activity was assayed in an aliquot of the cell suspension (A). Membrane fractions were isolated as described (8), and glucose transport was assayed in plasma membranes (B). The concentration of glucose transporters in plasma membranes (C) and in low-density microsomes (D) was determined with the cytochalasin B binding assay (8). The data represent means of three separate experiments. Cells were treated with KCN prior to homogenization in 2 experiments without any difference in the results.

DISCUSSION AND CONCLUSIONS

Extending previous findings obtained with the cytochalasin B binding assay, the present data indicate that isoproterenol inhibits glucose transport activity without altering the concentration of plasma membrane glucose transporters. Further, these data demonstrate specific changes in adipose cell protein phosphorylation in response to insulin and isoproterenol. In particular, the phosphorylation of several cytosolic proteins was enhanced under conditions which stimulated glucose transport (insulin incubation), and decreased when glucose transport activity was inhibited by isoproterenol. The data thus support the notion that insulin-induced protein phosphorylation is involved in mediating the metabolic effects of the hormones, possibly via an insulin-dependent kinase which is inhibited by catecholamines. However, the glucose transporter itself cannot be a target of this kinase, since its phosphorylation state remained unaltered when transport was stimulated by insulin or subsequently reduced by isoproterenol. Conversely, transporters were phosphorylated in response to phorbol ester without any change in either transporter activity or transporter translocation, indicating that their phosphorylation does not regulate the activity of glucose transport in the rat adipose cell. The present data confirm and extend the findings of a recent study on 3T3-L1 fatty fibroblasts in which no phosphate incorporation into the glucose transporter was detected in basal and insulin-stimulated cells (2).

Surprisingly, the cell fractionation employed in our study revealed that transporters phosphorylated in response to phorbol ester were located exclusively in the plasma membranes, and not in low-density microsomes. Thus, it is tempting to speculate that in the presence of maximally stimulating   insulin   concentrations,   the plasma   membrane   transporters equilibrate very slowly, if at all, with the intracellular pool.   Alternativley, phorbol ester might "lock" glucose transporters in the plasma membrane, possibly by their phosphorylation, and prevent their recycling into the low-density microsomes.

REFERENCES

1. Cushman, S.W., and Wardzala, L.J. (1980): *J. Biol. Chem.*, 255:4758-4762.
2. Gibbs, E.M., Allard, W.J., and Lienhard, G.E. (1986): *J. Biol. Chem.*, 261:16597-16603.
3. Haspel, H.C., Birnbaum, M.J., Wilk, E.W., and Rosen, O. M. (1985): *J. Biol. Chem.*, 260:7219-7225.
4. Joost, H.G., Weber, T.M., Cushman, S.W., and Simpson, I.A. (1986): *J. Biol. Chem.*, 261:10033-10036.
5. Joost, H.G., Weber, T.M., Cushman, S.W., and Simpson, I.A. (1987): *J. Biol. Chem.*, 262:11261-11267.
6. Rodbell, M. (1964): *J. Biol. Chem.*, 239:375-380.
7. Simpson, I.A., Yver, D.R., Hissin, P.J., Wardzala, L.J., Karnielli, E., Salans, L.B., Cushman, S.W. (1983): *Biochim. Biophys. Acta* 763:393-407.
8. Weber, T.M., Joost, H.G., Simpson, I.A., and Cushman, S.W. (1988): In: *Receptor Biochemistry and Methodology,* edited by C.R. Kahn and L.C. Harrison, (in press). Alan R. Liss, New York.
9. Wheeler, T.J., Simpson, I.A., Sogin, D.C., Hinkle, P.C., and Cushman, S.W. (1982): *Biochem. Biophys. Res. Commun.,* 105:89-95.

Insulin Action and Diabetes,
edited by H. Joseph Goren et al.
Raven Press, New York © 1988.

REGULATION OF HEXOSE TRANSPORTER PROTEIN EXPRESSION

Howard C. Haspel, Morris J. Birnbaum and Ora M. Rosen

Program of Molecular Biology
Memorial Sloan-Kettering Cancer Center
1275 York Avenue
New York, NY 10021

Glucose is passively transported into most mammalian cells. This process is energy dependent, stereospecific, and sensitive to inhibition by cytochalasin B (10,14,15). A 55 kD integral membrane glycoprotein has been shown to mediate this process (10,14,15). Three years ago we produced polyclonal rabbit antisera to the, purified human erythrocyte glucose transporter (α-GT) (5). α-GT specifically immunoblotted and immunoprecipitated hexose transporters from mammalian tissues and cultured cells. We used this antisera to describe the biosynthesis of the mammalian hexose transporter (5) and to clone a full length cDNA of the transporter from rat brain (1). Recently we have used α-GT and the cDNA to describe the regulation of hexose transporter expression in rodent fibroblasts by glucose deprivation (6) and cellular transformation (2).

HEXOSE TRANSPORTER BIOSYNTHESIS

The mammalian hexose transporter is derived from a primary translation product of apparent molecular weight (Mr) 38,000 (5). The same electrophoretic mobility is exhibited by the transporter after enzymatic deglycosylation <u>in vitro</u> or after tunicamycin treatment of intact cells (5). The primary translation product is cotranslationally core glycosylated to a Mr 42,000 membrane inserted precursor which subsequently "matures", via oligosaccharide "trimming", to the heterogeneously glycosylated transporter of Mr 50-60,000 (5).

163

Isolation of the full length cDNA of the rat brain hexose transporter allowed us to determine the nucleotide sequence of the cDNA encoding the transporter, and to deduce the amino acid sequence of the transporter protein (1). The nucleotide sequence of the rat glucose transporter cDNA is nearly identical (>85%) to that of the human glucose transporter (1,11). The deduced amino acid sequence of the rat transporter differs from that of the human transporter by only twelve amino acids and predicts a 56 kD polypeptide (1,11). A computer generated model of the transmembrane topology of the rat transporter is similar to that reported for the human transporter (1,11). The predictions made by this model include: twelve hydrophobic or amphipathic membrane spanning regions, cytoplasmically oriented carboxy- and amino-termini, lack of a cleavable signal sequence and a large cytoplasmically oriented hydrophilic loop in the middle of the polypeptide. The model also predicts that the more amino-terminal of two potential sites for N-linked oligosaccharide attachment is utilized (1,11).

EXPRESSION OF GLUCOSE TRANSPORTER PROTEIN AND mRNA IN DIFFERENT TISSUE AND CELL TYPES

The cDNA and α-GT allowed us to demonstrate that insulin-sensitive and insulin-insensitive hexose transporters are both derived from similar 2.8 kb mRNA's and Mr 38,000 core polypeptides (1). Surprisingly, aside from alterations due to glycosylation, the hexose transporters of most mammalian tissues and cells examined appeared quite similar (1,2,5,6,10,14,15). The abundance of the transporter protein and mRNA in "normal" (i.e., not transformed) tissues and cells is also similar (1). Whole brain tissue, however, has approximately five-fold more transporter protein and mRNA than cultured primary fibroblasts (1). An interesting exception to this constitutive level of expression was our finding that normal rat and human liver tissue, in contrast to hepatoma cells, contain very little if any of this transporter and must, therefore, express one or more immunologically and genetically distinct transporter(s) (1). Furthermore, Southern blots of rat and human DNA suggest that a single gene encodes the rat brain transporter (1).

REGULATION BY GLUCOSE DEPRIVATION

It is well known that glucose deprivation of cultured cells increases the Vmax for hexose transport by approximately five-fold (c.f. 16). The molecular mechanisms underlying this change were, however, not understood. We employed α-GT and the cDNA to examine this question in murine 3T3 fibroblasts (6). When the fibroblasts are deprived of glucose for 24-48 h they exhibit a five-fold increase in both hexose transport and cytochalasin B binding. Immunoblots of membranes of cells fed glucose (4 g/l) for 48 h reveal the M_r 55,000 transporter. Transporter proteins of a M_r 55,000 and M_r 42,000 are detected in cells deprived of glucose for 48 h. A ten- to forty-fold increase in total transporter protein occurs upon glucose deprivation; part of this accumulation (two- to five-fold) is in the M_r 55,000 form and the remaining increase is in the M_r 42,000 form. During the first 12 h of glucose deprivation only the M_r 55,000 form accumulates. At later times (24-72 h) the M_r 42,000 form appears and ultimately constitutes a large fraction of the total accumulation. The M_r 55,000 form accumulates when cells are incubated at higher concentrations of glucose (≤ 2 g/l) than the M_r 42,000 form (≤ 0.5 g/l).

Using alternative nutrients, sugar analogs, and inhibitors we observed that accumulation of total transporter is dependent upon **both** hexose phosphate metabolism and the interaction of substrate with the transporter. The roles of oligosaccharide biosynthesis, protein synthesis, and the transport process itself in the glucose deprivation-induced accumulation of transporter polypeptides were also examined. The appearance of the M_r 42,000 form, but not the accumulation of the M_r 55,000 form, was dependent upon protein synthesis. The accumulation of total transporters was not dependent upon protein glycosylation. The glucose deprivation-induced accumulation of transporter polypeptides was reversible upon refeeding with glucose (4 g/l) for 12 h. This reversal was also dependent upon protein synthesis. The electrophoretic mobility of the M_r 42,000 form is similar to the that observed after treatment of cells with tunicamycin. The M_r 55,000 form, but not the M_r 42,000 form, binds specifically to agarose-bound wheat germ agglutinin and is sensitive to endoglycosidase F digestion. Oligosaccharide-stripped transporter and the M_r 42,000 form have similar M_r's. These results suggest that the accumulation of total transporter which is induced by glucose deprivation is partially independent of the effect of glucose deprivation on glycoprotein biogenesis. The appearance of the M_r 42,000 form with "aglyco" characteristics is the result of the latter. The accumulation of total transporter, however, is the result of a specialized and sensitive adaptation of the cell to glucose deprivation. The M_r 42,000 form of the transporter is synthesized during chronic glucose deprivation while fed cells synthesize the M_r 55,000 form. The level of glucose transporter mRNA, in vitro translatable transporter mRNA, and the rate of transporter synthesis are **not** increased by glucose deprivation. It is likely, therefore, that the accumulation of transporters during glucose deprivation is the result of decreased degradation.

Elevation of glucose transport is an alteration common to most virally-induced tumors (c.f. 7,12). To address the molecular mechanisms underlying this well known phenomenon rat fibroblasts transformed with wild-type or a temperature-sensitive Fujinami sarcoma virus (FSV) were studied (2). FSV transforms cells by inducing the expression of the gag-fps tyrosine protein kinase (4). Five- to ten-fold increases in total cellular glucose transporter protein occurred in response to transformation by FSV and are accompanied by similar increases in transporter mRNA levels. These changes were observed as early as 2 h after placing cells at the permissive temperature for transformation and plateaued at 24 h. An absolute increase in the rate of glucose transporter gene transcription occurred within 30 min after the temperature was shifted to induce transformation. The transporter mRNA levels in transformed fibroblasts were higher than those found in "normal" proliferating cells which, in turn, were higher than those of confluent cells maintained at the nonpermissive temperature. Transformation of fibroblasts by the src and ras, but not the myc oncogenes has also been shown to increase the level of transporter protein and mRNA (3). Serum (8), phorbol esters (3), and tumor necrosis factor (9) have also been shown to have similar effects. Although, alterations in glucose transporter degradation and/or processing may contribute (13) to the enhanced transport characteristic of transformed cells, it is likely that most of the increase in transporter protein observed upon oncogenic transformation, in the systems examined, is attributable to increased transporter biosynthesis. The activation of transporter gene transcription by transformation represents one of the earliest known effects of oncogenesis on the expression of a gene encoding a protein with a well defined function. The relative contributions of oncogenesis and growth to this phenomenon remain to be resolved.

SUMMARY

We have demonstrated that the primary protein structure of the glucose transporter is highly conserved between rats and humans (1). The transporter in cells exhibiting both insulin-sensitive and insulin-insensitive hexose transport is derived from a single M_r 38,000 primary translation product encoded by a single 2.8 kb mRNA (1, 5). The rat brain transporter is constitutively expressed at similar levels in all tissues examined except for liver and brain (1). Brain has five-fold higher levels of transporter protein and mRNA than most other tissues whereas normal liver has very little, if any (1). It is likely, therefore, that other immunologically and genetically distinct kinds of hexose transporters will be found in hepatocytes and perhaps other cell types.

We have found that glucose deprivation of fibroblasts leads to increased glucose transport by stabilizing the transporter protein (6). This process is regulated by the presence of **both** hexose phosphates and substrate for the transporter (6). On the other hand, oncogenic transformation of mammalian fibroblasts leads to increased glucose transport mainly by increasing the rate of transcription of the glucose transporter gene (2,3). Cell proliferation alone increases the level of transporter mRNA but does not completely account for the marked changes observed upon oncogenic transformation (2,3).

In conclusion there are at least three independent mechanisms for activating glucose transport in mammalian cells: increasing the half-life of the glucose transporter protein (6,13,16), intrinsic activation and/or translocation of existing glucose transporters (10,14,14), and stimulation of glucose transporter synthesis (2,3,13). Examples of physiologically relevant changes which fall into each of these three categories are glucose deprivation (2,13,16), acute insulin stimulation (10,14,15), and cellular transformation (2,3,13), respectively.

REFERENCES

1. Birnbaum, M.J., Haspel, H.C., and Rosen, O.M. (1986): **Proc. Natl. Acad. Sci. USA**, 83:5784-5788.

2. Birnbaum, M.J., Haspel, H.C., and Rosen, O.M. (1987): **Science**, 235:1495-1498.

3. Flier, J.S., Mueckler, M.M., Usher, P., and Lodish, H.F. (1987): **Science**, 235:1492-1495.

4. Hanufusa, T., Mathey-Provot, B., Feldman, R.A., and Hanufusa, H. (1981): **J. Virol.**, 38:347-354.

5. Haspel, H.C., Birnbaum, M.J., Wilk. E.W., and Rosen, O.M. (1985): **J. Biol. Chem.**, 260:7219-7225.

6. Haspel, H.C., Wilk, E.W., Birnbaum, M.J., Cushman, S.W., and Rosen, O.M. (1986): **J. Biol. Chem.**, 261:6778-6789.

7. Kawai, S., and Hanufusa, H. (1971): **Virology**, 46:470-479.

8. Kletzien, R.F., and Purdue, S.K. (1974): **J. Biol. Chem.**, 249:3366-3387.

9. Lee, M.D., Zentella, A., Pekela, P.H., and Cerami, A.
    (1987): **Proc. Natl. Acad. Sci. USA**, 84:2590-2594.

10. Lienhard, G.E. (1983): **Trends Biochem. Sci.**, 8:125-127.

11. Mueckler, M., Caruso, C., Baldwin, S.A., Panico, M.,
    Blench, I., Morris, H.R., Allard, W.J., Lienhard, G.E, and
    Lodish, H.F. (1985): **Science**, 229:941-945.

12. Salter, D.W., Baldwin, S.A., Lienhard, G.E., and Weber,
    M.J. (1982): **Proc. Natl. Acad. Sci. USA**, 79:1540-1544.

13. Shawver, L.K., Olson, S.A., White, M.K., and Weber, M.J.
    (1987): **Mol. Cell. Biol.**, 7:2112-2118.

14. Simpson, I.A., and Cushman, S.W. (1986): **Ann. Rev.
    Biochem.**, 55:1059-1089.

15. Wheeler, T.J., and Hinkle, P.C. (1985): **Ann. Rev.
    Physiol.**, 47:503-517.

16. Yamada, K., Tillotson, L.G., and Isselbacher, K.J.
    (1983): **J. Biol. Chem.**, 258:9786-9792.

Insulin Action and Diabetes,
edited by H. Joseph Goren et al.
Raven Press, New York © 1988.

REGULATION OF S6 PROTEIN KINASE FROM HUMAN PLACENTA: EVIDENCE FOR ACTIVATION BY AN ACTIVATING ENZYME AND THE INSULIN RECEPTOR

Ruthann A. Masaracchia, Sushanta Mallick, and Fern E. Murdoch

Department of Biochemistry
University of North Texas
Denton, Texas 76202

The S6 protein in the 40S ribosome is multi-phosphorylated in insulin-treated cells. Several reports of S6 kinases have appeared in the literature. In this laboratory we have used human placenta as a source for the isolation and characterization of S6 kinases. In the course of these experiments an activating enzyme for the S6 kinase has been identified (1,2). In this report the regulation of the S6 kinase and the activating enzyme (AE) by the insulin receptor is described.

A gel filtration profile which is the last step in a purification scheme for S6 kinase from human placenta is shown in FIG. 1. An S6 kinase activity which is activated by MgATP elutes with an Mr 85,000. This enzyme is analogous to that previously isolated from lymphosarcoma cells (4). In addition to catalyzing multisite phosphorylation of S6 in the 40S ribosome (3), the enzyme phosphorylates histone H4 and a synthetic peptide derived from one of the S6 phosphorylation sites (RRLSSLRA). A prominent phosphoprotein with Mr 55,000 coincides with the elution of the MgATP-activated S6 kinase activity.

A second S6 kinase occurs as an inactive enzyme. This enzyme can be activated by brief digestion with 0.1% trypsin. If the MgATP-activated S6 kinase activity is subtracted from the total S6 kinase activity observed after trypsin-activation, the Mr of the latent S6 kinase is 158,000. This activity coincides with the elution of proteins with Mr 95,000 and 55,000 in a 1:1 stoichiometry, as determined by SDS PAGE.

In addition to the S6 kinases, a third enzyme activity in this elution profile has been detected (FIG.1). When a fraction (#65) obtained from the S6 kinase portion of the elution profile is incubated with MgATP and aliquots from fractions 50-59, biphasic activation of the S6 kinase is observed. The first AE fractions elute with the void volume; the second AE activity elutes just prior to the trypsin-sensitive S6 kinase.

In order to further investigate this AE, monoclonal antibodies

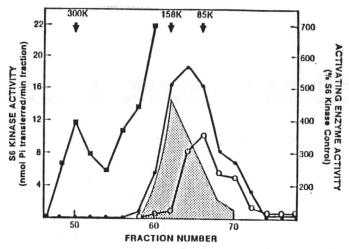

FIG. 1. Elution from Sephacryl S200 of S6 kinase activity and activating enzyme from human placenta. Enzyme obtained from DEAE and phosphocellulose chromatrography was eluted from a Sephacryl S200 column (100x2.5 cm) in 3.6 ml fractions. S6 kinase activity was determined subsequent to MgATP activation(-O-) or trypsin activation(-●-). AE activity(-□-) was determined in the presence of 5 μl from fraction 65. The shaded area is net trypsin-dependent S6 kinase activity.

to AE were prepared. Purification of AE by monoclonal antibody affinity chromatrography demonstrated that this enzyme contained two subunits with Mr 116,000 and 72,000 (FIG. 2). When the purified AE is added to the S6 kinases, activation of those enzymes (not shown) and phosphorylation of the 95,000 and 55,000 proteins are enhanced (FIG. 3). No autophosphorylation of the AE is observed.

Some Mr 72,000 also elutes with the MgATP-activated S6 kinase as determined by ELISA, and it is postulated that this is the endogenous activating enzyme. In confirmation, the removal of the Mr 72,000 protein from the S6 kinase preparation with a monoclonal antibody also prevented S6 kinase activation, although the S6 kinase was not removed by the antibody (Table 1).

TABLE 1. Removal of Mr 72k protein in the S6 kinase preparation.

S6 Kinase Treatment[a]	S6 Kinase Activity (pmol/min)	
	-activation	+activation
Control, initial	1.1	18
Control, assayed in wells	1.5	8.3
Antip72 antibody-treated	0.7	3.9

[a]Cell culture wells were coated with rabbit antimouse IgG and antip72 monoclonal IgG (5) and incubated 10 min with S6 kinase prior to MgATP activation and assay with H4.

Our hypothesis is that the 72,000 subunit is the catalytic subunit of the AE and the 116,000 subunit is the regulatory protein. To investigate the potential regulation of AE by growth factor, AE and insulin receptor (kindly provided by Richard Roth, Stanford University) were incubated with MgATP and the proteins were analyzed by SDS PAGE and autoradiography (FIG. 4).

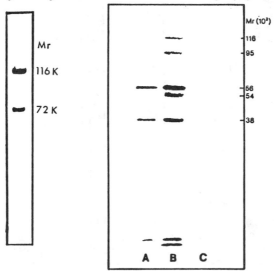

FIG. 2. AE purified by antibody affinity chromatography (left). FIG. 3. Phosphorylation of Mr 95,000 and 55,000 proteins in the S6 kinase preparations by AE. S6 kinase alone(A) or with AE(B) or AE(C) alone was incubated with Mg[γ-^{32}P]ATP for 10 min and phosphoproteins analyzed by SDS PAGE and autoradiography (shown).

The insulin receptor catalyzed phosphorylation of the Mr 116,000 subunit of the antibody-purified AE (FIG. 4). We previously demonstrated that the insulin receptor also enhanced phosphorylation of the Mr 95,000 protein in a preparation of S6 kinases containing both AE and S6 kinase (6).   In Table 2 the effect of the insulin receptor on S6 kinase activity was investigated.   No effect of the insulin receptor on the AE or S6 kinase activity alone was observed. By contrast, when the AE and the S6 kinases were incubated together with the insulin receptor, enhancement of both H4 and S6 peptide phosphorylation was observed.
In summary, the data are consistent with the hypothesis that there is a phosphorylation cascade which can mediate intracellular events initiated by insulin activation of the insulin receptor tyrosine kinase and that this cascade includes both the S6 kinase(s) and an intermediary enzyme, AE.

ACKNOWLEDGMENTS

This work was supported in part by grant GM 32350 from the NIH and grant 186222 from the Juvenile Diabetes Foundation.

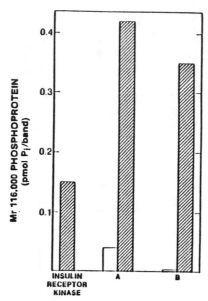

FIG. 4.   Phosphorylation of the Mr 116,000 subunit of the AE by the insulin receptor. AE was incubated alone (open bars) or with insulin receptor (shaded bars) and MgATP. Proteins were analyzed by SDS PAGE and phospho-116 protein was quantitated by liquid scintillation counting of the excised band.

TABLE 2.   Activation of S6 kinase activity by insulin receptor.

Enzyme	S6 kinase activity (pmol/min)			
	RRLSSLRA		H4	
	-IR	+IR	-IR	+IR
AE	<0.2	<0.2	<0.2	<0.2
S6 Kinase	2.0	3.0	16	15
AE + S6 kinase	2.0	16	16	52

REFERENCES

1. de la Houssaye, B. A., Eckols, T.K., and Masaracchia, R. A. (1983) J. Biol. Chem. **258**:4272-4278.
2. de la Houssaye, B. A., Murdoch, F. E., and Masaracchia, R. A. (1988) J. Biol. Chem. In press.
3. Donahue, M. J. and Masaracchia, R. A. (1984) J. Biol. Chem. **259**:435-440.
4. Masaracchia, R. A., Kemp, B. E. and Walsh, D. A. (1977) J. Biol. Chem. **252**:7109-7117.
5. Morgan, D. O. and Roth, R. A. (1985) Endocrinology **116**:1224-1226.
6. Roth, R. A., Morgan, D. O. and Masaracchia, R. A. (1985) Cancer Cells **3**:109-113.

Insulin Action and Diabetes,
edited by H. Joseph Goren et al.
Raven Press, New York © 1988.

STUDIES ON THE REGULATION OF ACETYL–CoA
CARBOXYLASE BY INSULIN

Roger W. Brownsey, Katherine A. Quayle, and Alice L–F. Mui

Department of Biochemistry
University of British Columbia
2146 Health Sciences Mall
Vancouver, British Columbia
Canada   V6T 1W5

INTRODUCTION

In this symposium a strong emphasis has been placed on events which occur rapidly upon binding of insulin to its cell surface receptors. In particular, proteins located within the plasma membrane and events taking place within (or within very close proximity to) the same membrane have been highlighted, including the structure and activity of the insulin receptor and of the glucose transporter. This essay is concerned with the mechanisms by which the effects of insulin may be expressed as increased activity of the intracellular enzyme acetyl–CoA carboxylase.

The pathway for the conversion of glucose into long–chain fatty acids exhibits several points at which the flow of carbon may be regulated in response to altered nutritional status of the whole animal or in response to acute changes in hormone concentration in vivo or experimentally. This discussion will be concerned with the acute regulation of one of these key regulatory proteins. The structure and regulation of the glucose transport system is described in detail elsewhere in this volume. A detailed description of other key enzymes including phosphofructo–1–kinase, pyruvate kinase and the mitochondrial pyruvate dehydrogenase complex is beyond the scope of this article.

The control of the activity of acetyl–CoA carboxylase plays a major role in the regulation of de novo fatty acid biosynthesis in mammalian adipose tissue and liver and probably also in the mammalian gland. The expression of acetyl–CoA carboxylase may be regulated through changes in rates of protein synthesis and or degradation (with a half–time of the order of many hours) in response to hormones and nutritional status. In addition, the specific activity of acetyl-CoA carboxylase may be altered within a few minutes following exposure of intact tissue to insulin (which leads to activation) or to hormones which increase intracellular cyclic AMP concentrations and which lead to inhibition. Since the first description of acetyl-CoA carboxylase by Wakil and coworkers (41) a large number of studies have contributed to a rather detailed investigation of the structure, function and regulation of the enzyme. For a detailed account and for extensive bibliography the reader is referred to several recent reviews (8,18,24,31, 42,44). The view of the hormone-mediated regulation of acetyl-CoA carboxylase which has emerged from these studies is complex and still somewhat fragmentary. It seems reasonable to conclude that two broad topics must be considered for an integrated view − regulation through hormone-directed protein phosphorylation and dephosphorylation as well as allosteric regulation by small (or perhaps large) molecular weight modulators.

ROLE OF REVERSIBLE PHOSPHORYLATION IN RESPONSES TO INSULIN

Detailed studies of the proteins which exhibit altered activity in response to insulin have revealed that many of these target proteins demonstrate rapidly reversible phosphorylation catalyzed by protein kinases and protein phoshatases (2,10,16,33). Furthermore, changes in the extent of phosphorylation of these proteins may direclty or indirectly lead to changes in activity within intact cells and in purified systems (see several sections of 16,33). Reversible protein phosphorylation may therefore offer a general intracellular mechanism to account for many of the short-term (and perhaps longer term) effects of insulin on cell metabolism. However, there are many complexities within this broad mechanism to account for the direct actions of insulin (which involve both increases and decreases in specific protein phosphorylation) and also less direct actions which are most apparent following prior treatment with other hormones.

INSULIN PROMOTES INCREASES AND DECREASES
IN SPECIFIC PROTEIN PHOSPHORYLATION

Studies on the regulation of several well-characterized proteins have revealed that changes in activity in response to insulin treatment of tissue are associated with net dephosphorylation, and examples include enzymes activated by insulin such as pyruvate dehydrogenase (26) and glycogen synthase (32) and also enzymes which become less active in response to insulin including triacylglycerol lipase (30). In the case of the hormone-sensitive lipase, the observed dephosphorylation (of a single site) is only apparent after prior phosphorylation and activation by cyclic AMP-dependent protein kinase (39).

However, the activation of pyruvate dehydrogenase or glycogen synthase is more complex since phosphorylation occurs at multiple sites and requires cyclic AMP-independent protein kinases which are intramitochondrial and cytoplasmic respectively. Furthermore, it has been recognized that there exists a family of proteins which exhibit increases in phosphorylation in response to insulin treatment of tissues (2,10). In adipose tissue examples of proteins which become more highly phosphorylated in response to insulin include ATP-citrate lyase (1), acetyl-CoA carboxylase (7,13,43), the ribosomal protein S6 (37) and proteins so far only identified according to their subunit M_r of 22,000 and 61,000 (3,4). All except the latter two have also been identified in liver cells where the most striking response to insulin is the increased phosphorylation of an additional protein of subunit M_r 46,000 (25). Most recently the increased phosphorylation of the ß-subunit of the insulin receptor in response to insulin treatment has been demonstrated in a number of cell types and with isolated receptors incubated in vitro (see several chapters in this volume).

TABLE 1. Proteins exhibiting changes in phosphorylation in fat cells exposed to insulin

Decreases in phosphorylation	Increases in phosphorylation
Pyruvate dehydrogenase (α-subunit)	Acetyl CoA carboxylase
Triglyceride lipase[a]	ATP citrate lyase
Glycogen phosphorylase[a]	Insulin receptor (ß-subunit)
Phosphorylase[a]	Ribosomal S_6 protein
Glycogen synthase	61 K plasma-membrane protein
	22 K cytoplsmic protein (heat/acid stable)

[a] Effects most apparent after treatment of tissues with hormones which increase cellular cyclic AMP.

Since the demonstration that acetyl-CoA carboxylase becomes phosphorylated within intact fat cells (13) it has been found that the activation of the enzyme in response to insulin (7,13, 43) and also the inhibition observed following incubation of fat cells with adrenaline (12) are both accompanied by modest overall increases in phosphorylation of the enzyme. The explanation of this apparent paradox came with the demonstration that acetyl-CoA carboxylase was phosphorylated at multiple sites (19) and that insulin and adrenaline essentially brought about phosphorylation of different sites. The activation of acetyl-CoA carboxylase in response to insulin is accompanied by phosphorylation of at least one serine residue located on a tryptic peptide (designated as the I-peptide) which may be separated by two-dimensional mapping from peptides (A-peptides) which show increased phosphorylation in response to adrenaline (7). The effects of adrenaline or glucagon are mimicked in vitro by incubation of purified acetyl-CoA carboxylase with the catalytic subunit of cyclic AMP-dependent protein kinase (19) apparently with phosphorylation of the same peptides (9,19). Independent studies have also demonstrated the effect of insulin on the phosphorylation of acetyl-CoA carboxylase within fat cells (21,45) and liver cells (43,47). In addition, using HPLC to separate phosphopeptides it has been shown that the phosphorylation of acetyl-CoA carboxylase within liver cells (23) and fat cells (22) in response to glucagon is probably catalyzed by cyclic AMP-dependent protein kinase.

EFFECTS OF PHOSPHORYLATION ON THE ACTIVITY OF ACETYL-CoA CARBOXYLASE

Most studies have concentrated on the effects of phosphorylation of acetyl-CoA carboxylase in the presence of the catalytic subunit of cyclic AMP-dependent protein kinase. This treatment leads to reduced activity of highly purified preparations of acetyl-CoA carboxylase which may be observed at low or at high concentrations of the allosteric activator citrate. This treatment with free catalytic subunit of protein kinase produces changes in the properties of acetyl-CoA carboxylase which are very similar to those observed following treatment of intact fat cells with adrenaline or glucagon (12,22) or treatment of liver cells with glucagon (23). The inhibition of acetyl-CoA carboxylase seen in intact cells (12) or in vitro (19) are reversed upon treatment with protein phosphatases. Furthermore, peptide analysis by HPLC or by two-dimensional mapping has revealed that the phosphorylation of acetyl-CoA carboxylase in the presence of cyclic AMP-dependent protein kinase occurs at sites apparently identical to those occupied on the enzyme isolated from intact cells treated with adrenaline or glucagon (9,22,23). These studies offer convincing support for the hypothesis that the effects of adrenaline or glucagon (which bring about inhibition of acetyl-CoA carboxylase) are mediated by cyclic AMP-dependent protein kinase. One aspect perhaps not fully explored is that the effects observed in vitro are much slower than those observed within intact cells.

Studies of insulin-directed phosphorylation of acetyl-CoA carboxylase have progressed more slowly because purified preparations of the protein kinases and protein phosphatases involved have not so far been available. Progress has been facilitated by the observation that insulin-stimulated protein serine kinase activity may be detected in subcellular fractions following the exposure of intact cells to the hormone. This has allowed some characterization of this activity (or activities) in extracts from 3T3-L1 cells (14,15) from rat epididymal adipose tissue (11) and from hepatoma cells (29). These different studies all confirm that insulin-stimulated activity of protein kinase differs from some well-characterized activities being independent of cyclic nucleotides, calcium ions, phospholipid plus diacylglycerol or proteolytic activation. Nevertheless, the studies still reveal substantial differences in properties of insulin-stimulated protein kinase in the different cells even when a common substrate (the ribosmal protein S6) has been employed (14,15,29). These differences in properties may indicate rather subtle inter-tissue variation but could also indicate that more than one protein kinase is activated in response to insulin. The true nature of the complexities involved will require much further work but exciting progress seems imminent with two very recent reports which provide more extensive characterization and purification of S6 kinases (see 40 and also the report of Dr. Masaraccio in the proceedings of this symposium). It will clearly be important to establish the extent to which these S6-kinases are able to phosphorylate other proteins which show increased phosphorylation in response to insulin including acetyl-CoA carboxylase.

EFFECTS OF INSULIN ON THE ACTIVITY OF ACETYL-CoA CARBOXYLASE

Activation of acetyl-CoA carboxylase in response to insulin has been observed in white (38) and brown adipose tissue (27), in liver (38) and in mammary gland (28) in vivo; and with intact adipose tissue (17) or isolated fat (6) or liver cells (46) in vitro. In fat and liver a good correspondence has been observed between rates of fatty acid synthesis (followed by incorporation of labelled precursors) and the proportion of acetyl-CoA carboxylase in the active (presumably polymeric) form detected subsequently in tissue supernatant fractions. Activity of acetyl-CoA carboxylase has been determined immediately upon extraction ("initial" activity) and then expressed as a proportion of the activity measured following exposure in vitro to maximally-activating concentrations of citrate and of defatted serum albumin ("total" activity). Insulin promotes an increase in activity of acetyl-CoA carboxylase observed at low (physiological) concentrations of added citrate in the range 0-1 mM. The effects of insulin, unlike the effects of adrenaline or glucagon, are abolished by incubation of acetyl-CoA carboxylase in the presence of high concentrations of citrate.

Since it was initially anticipated that the activity of acetyl-CoA carboxylase would be dictated by the balance between binding of activating and inhibitory allosteric effectors, it was surprising that the altered activity could be detected even after dilution of the intracellular cytosolic fraction by as much as several-hundred fold.

The activity of acetyl-CoA carboxylase in purified or freshly extracted preparations may be altered in vitro by physiological concentrations of a number of small molecular weight ligands including citrate, fatty acyl-SCoA esters, guanine nucleotides, free Coenzyme A, polyamines and phospholipids (for reviews, see 8,24). In general, the effects of ligands are reflected by changes in activity and parallel changes in the equilibrium between the protomeric form of the enzyme with low specific activity (dimers of M_r approximately 500,000) and more active polymeric forms (with M_r in the range 5-10 X 10^6). Despite the in vitro observations, it has been a complex problem to elucidate the extent to which the different ligands may influence the activity and degree of polymerization of acetyl-CoA carboxylase within intact cells. Many studies have attempted to relate acetyl-CoA carboxylase activity to observed tissue concentrations of proposed effectors (for review, see 8). The relationship between tissue concentrations of citrate and the degree of activation of acetyl-CoA carboxylase is certainly difficult to discern. Thus incubation of tissues in the presence of insulin leads to little or no change in citrate concentrations. In contrast, striking increases in whole tissue citrate (5-20 fold) are observed upon incubation of adipose tissue in the presence of pyruvate, hydroxycitrate or fluoroacetate with no corresponding changes in acetyl-CoA carboxylase activity. Perhaps more convincing evidence would support the contention that the tissue cocentration of fatty acyl CoA esters is inversely related to acetyl-CoA carboxylase activity. Even so, such whole tissue determinations of metabolic intermediates can take little account of distribution between different subcellular compartments or (perhaps equally important) of the distribution between aqueous and hydrophobic phases or between free and bound forms. In summary, there is little convincing evidence that changes in activity of acetyl-CoA carboxylase in response to insulin or to other hormones may be adequately explained by changes in the concentrations of potentially regulatory allosteric ligands.

The deductions drawn from measurement of tissue cocentrations of potential regulators of acetyl-CoA carboxylase are supported by further evidence concerning the persistence of the hormone effects with different treaments of the enzyme following tissue extraction. The first indication of this phenomenon was persistence of activation of acetyl-CoA carboxylase following tissue homogenization. It has further been shown that the effects of hormones on acetyl-CoA carboxylase are still apparent after purification through ammonium sulfate precipitation with subsequent resuspension and dialysis and also following sedimentation in the presence of citrate (7). Further evidence has shown activation in response to insulin is still apparent after purification of acetyl–CoA carboxylase by FPLC on Superose columns (5). One recent report (20) has suggested that the effects of insulin on the activity of acetyl–CoA carboxylase may be abolished by subjecting the enzyme to chromatography over size exclusion columns after exposure to high concentrations of salt. However, we have been unable to find similar abolition of the effects of insulin. In five separate experiments the activation of acetyl–CoA carboxylase in response to insulin was initially 168±7% of control and following incubation in the presence of KCl (0.5 M) and subsequent rapid gel filtration over G–25 sephadex the observed activation was 163±5% control. The most extensive purification of acetyl–CoA carboxylase involving affinity chromatography employing avidin-sepharose has shown that the effects of glucagon but not the effects of insulin are still detected in the highly purified enzyme (21–23,47). In summarizing the above observations it seems reasonable to conclude that the effects of hormones on the activity of acetyl–CoA carboxylase are most unlikely to be explained by residual binding of readily dissociable ligands and that in the case of inhibition brought about by adrenaline or glucagon the phosphorylation may be necessary and sufficient for inhibition of the enzyme.

Since the effects of insulin appear to be lost with purification of acetyl–CoA carboxylase to homogeneity, it must remain a possibility that phosphorylation alone is not sufficient to bring about insulin–like activation. A difficult problem to resolve is that a hydrophobic ligand (or other ligand with very high affinity) may remain associated during extraction and further purification – to be removed only during the exacting conditions of affinity chromatography in the presence of 0.5 M KCl. A likely (although by no means the only) candidate for especially tight association with acetyl–CoA carboxylase may be long–chain acyl–CoA esters. Alternative possibilities which may be considered are less defined insulin "mediators" including the recently described product of hydrolytic cleavage of a novel glycolipid (35,36) which may perhaps be related to material previously reported to activate acetyl–CoA carboxylase (34). With incomplete description of these mediator preparations available at the present time it is not possible to predict if they would possess sufficiently high affinity for acetyl–CoA carboxylase to explain the observed persistence of the effects of insulin.

In order to address the possibility that residual binding of fatty acyl–CoA esters to acetyl–CoA carboxylase may explain the effects of insulin on the enzyme we have carried out the experiments illustrated in Figures 1–3. The first experiments involved addition of palmitoyl–CoA to fresh supernatant fractions from rat epididymal adipose tissue following exposure of

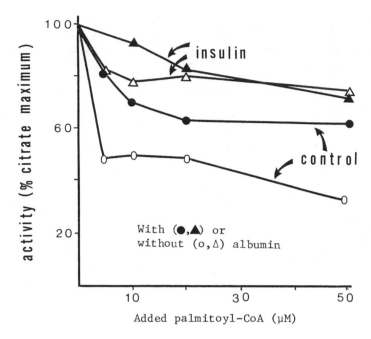

FIG. 1.   Effects of palmitoyl-CoA on acetyl-CoA
carboxylase activity in adipose tissue extracts.

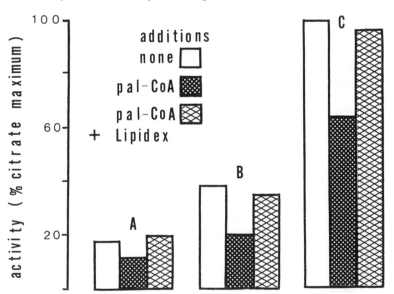

FIG. 2.   Effects of added palmitoyl-CoA on acetyl-CoA
carboxylase are reversed by Lipidex treatment.   In
panels A,B,C, citrate was added at 0, 0.5 or 10 mM

the intact tissue to insulin or no hormone. The added concentration of palmitoyl-CoA is reported but it must be stressed that the free concentration of the ligand available to acetyl-CoA carboxylase is likely to be substantially lower. The additions of acyl-CoA were made for only 2-5 min following the prior activation of acetyl-CoA carboxylase in the presence of 10 mM citrate. Substantial inhibition is observed and this is particularly marked in extracts from control (non insulin-treated) tissue. The effects of palmitoyl-CoA are reduced but not abolished by inclusion of defatted serum albumin. Subsequently, we have observed that the effects of palmitoyl-CoA may be reversed by treatment of extracts with lipophilic sephadex (LH-20, also commercially described as "Lipidex"). This matrix has been previously used by others to ensure delipidation of lipophilic ligand-binding proteins including serum albumin and fatty acid-binding protein. Results in Figure 2 illustrate that the inhibition of acetyl-CoA carboxylase is apparent at several tested concentrations of added citrate and in all cases the inhibition is reversed by the treatment with Lipidex. Although

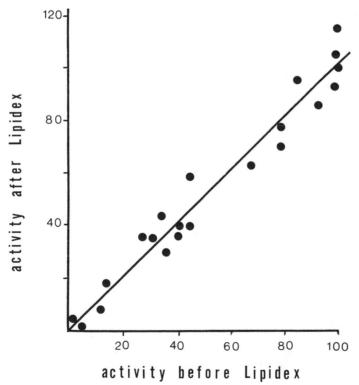

FIG. 3. Activity of acetyl-CoA carboxylase in fresh extracts of adipose tissue is unaffected by endogenous hydrophobic ligands.

the effects of added palmitoyl–CoA on acetyl–CoA carboxylase activity could be reversed by exposure to Lipidex, the exposure of extracts of adipose tissue to Lipidex alone results in no apparent change in enzyme activity. The results illustrated in Figure 3 includes a wide range of activities of acetyl–CoA carboxylase observed in extracts of tissue exposed to insulin or no hormone assayed with no prior exposure in vitro to citrate ("initial" activity) and also after partial activation or maximal activation with added citrate (at 1 mM or 10 mM respectively).

We conclude from these experiments that the effects of insulin on the activity of acetyl–CoA carboxylase observed in tissue extracts is most unlikely to be explained by altered binding of long–chain acyl–CoA esters or other hydrophobic ligands. Indeed the addition of near–physiological concentrations of palmitoyl–CoA actually exposes the effects of insulin when this has been masked by incubation in vitro in the presence of citrate.

CONCLUDING REMARKS

The rapid regulation of acetyl–CoA carboxylase in response to treatment of tissue with insulin continues to present an intriguing problem which is still not fully resolved. We appear to have a good understanding of a number of factors which are likely to be involved in the effects of insulin but still we do not have a clear appreciation of the mechanisms which operate within intact cells. Insulin–directed and site–specific phosphorylation of acetyl–CoA carboxylase may not be sufficient to account for the activation of the enzyme in response to insulin. Yet the persistence of the insulin–promoted activation suggests that the binding of classical allosteric ligand also is unlikely to completely explain the effects of the hormone. Perhaps some as yet untested combination of these two influences will reveal the true nature of the effect of insulin but equally plausible must be the possibility of unrecognized factors. Our own studies lead us to speculate that some protein–protein interaction may play a significant role since in combination with the requirement for a permissive phosphorylation of acetyl–CoA carboxylase this would explain a number of the observations described above. An additional attraction to maintaining a committed interest (dare I say persistent interest) in this problem is the hope that an understanding may prove to have a wider significance in our view of the possible physiological significance of phosphorylation of other proteins which exhibit increased phosphorylation in response to insulin.

ACKNOWLEDGEMENTS

We would like to express our thanks to the Julia Macfarlane Diabetes Foundation and other sponsors for making this symposium possible; to the meeting organizers and editors of this volume for giving us the opportunity to describe our studies and most importantly to the Medical Research Council of Canada and to the British Columbia Research Foundation for financial support.

REFERENCES

1. Alexander, M.C., Kowaloff, E.M., Witters, L.A, Dennihy, D.T. and Avruch, J. (1979): J. Biol. Chem., 254:8052-8056.
2. Avruch, J., Alexander, M.C., Palmer, J.L., Pierce, M.W., Nemenoff, R.A., Tipper, J.P. and Witters, L.A. (1982): Fed. Proc., 41:2629-2633.
3. Belsham, G.J. and Denton, R.M. (1980): Biochem. Soc. Trans., 8:382-383.
4. Belsham, G.J., Denton, R.M. and Tanner, M.J.A. (1980): Biochem. J., 192:457-467.
5. Borthwick, A.C., Edgell, N.J. and Denton, R.M. (1987): Biochem. J., 241:773-782.
6. Brownsey, R.W. (1983): Hormones and Cell Regulation, 7:85-102.
7. Brownsey, R.W. and Denton, R.M. (1982): Biochem. J., 202:77-86.
8. Brownsey, R.W. and Denton, R.M. (1987): In: The Enzymes, 3rd ed., vol. 18, pp. 123-146.
9. Brownsey, R.W. and Hardie, D.G. (1980): FEBS Lett., 120:67-70.
10. Brownsey, R.W., Denton, P.M. and Belsham, G.J. (1981): Diabetologia, 21:347-362.
11. Brownsey, R.W., Edgell, N.J., Hopkirk, T.J. and Denton, R.M. (1984): Biochem. J., 218:733-744.
12. Brownsey, R.W., Hughes, W.A. and Denton, R.M. (1979): Biochem. J., 184:23-32.
13. Brownsey, R.W., Hughes, W.A., Denton, R.M. and Mayer, R.J. (1977): Biochem. J., 168:441-445.
14. Cobb, M.H. (1986): J. Biol. Chem., 261:12984-12999.
15. Cobb, M.H. and Rosen, O.M. (1983): J. Biol. Chem., 258:12472-12481.
16. Czech, M.P., editor (1985): Molecular Basis of Insulin Action. Plenum Press, New York.
17. Halestrap, A.P. and Denton, R.M. (1973): Biochem. J., 132:509-517.
18. Hardie, D.G. (1980): In: Recently Discovered Systems of Enzyme Regulation by Reversible Phosphorylation, edited by P. Cohen, pp. 33-62. Elsevier Press, Amsterdam.
19. Hardie, D.G. and Guy, P.S. (1980): Eur. J. Biochem., 110:167-177.
20. Haystead, T.A.J. and Hardie, D.G. (1986): Biochem. J., 240:99-106.
21. Holland, R. and Hardie, D.G. (1985): FEBS Lett., 181:308-312.

22. Holland, R., Hardie, D.G., Clegg, R.A. and Zammit, V.A.
     (1985): Biochem. J., 226:139-149.
23. Holland, R., Witters, L.A. and Hardie, D.G. (1984): Eur.
     J. Biochem., 140:325-333.
24. Kim, K.-H. (1983): Curr. Top. Cell. Regul., 22:143-176.
25. LeCam, A. (1982): J. Biol. Chem., 257:8376-8385.
26. Martin, B.R., Denton, R.M., Pask, H. and Pandle, P.J.
     (1972): Biochem. J., 129:763-773.
27. McCormack, J.G. and Denton, R.M. (1977): Biochem. J.,
     166:627-630.
28. Munday, M.R. and Williamson, D.H. (1987): Biochem J.,
     242:905-911.
29. Nemenoff, R.A., Gunsalus, J.R. and Avruch, J. (1986):
     Arch. Bioch. Biophys., 245:106-203.
30. Nillson, N.O., Stralfors, P., Fredrickson, G. and
     Belfrage, P. (1980): FEBS Lett., 111:125-130.
31. Numa, S. and Tanabe, T. (1984): In: Fatty Acid Metabolism
     and Its Regulation, pp. 1-26. Elsevier Press, Amsterdam.
32. Parker, P.J., Caudwell,F.B. and Cohen, P. (1983): Eur. J.
     Biochem., 130:227-234.
33. Rosen, O.M. and Krebs, F.G., editors (1981): Protein
     Phosphorylation, Cold Spring Harbour Laboratory.
34. Saltiel, A.R., Doble, A., Jacobs, S. and Cuatrecasas, P.
     (1983): Biochem. Biophys. Res. Commun., 110:780-795.
35. Saltiel, A.R., Fox, J.A., Sherline, P. and Cuatrecasas, P.
     (1986): Science, 233:967-970.
36. Saltiel, A.R., Sherline, P. and Fox, J.A. (1987): J. Biol.
     Chem., 262:1116-1121.
37. Smith, C.J., Rubin, C.S. and Rosen, O.M. (1980): Proc.
     Natl. Acad. Sci., 77:2641-2645.
38. Stansbie, D., Brownsey, R.W., Crettaz, M. and Denton, R.M.
     (1976): Biochem. J., 160:413-416.
39. Stralfors, P. and Belfrage, P. (1983): J. Biol. Chem.,
     258:15146-15152.
40. Tabarini, D., de Herreros, A.G., Heinrich, J. and Rosen,
     O.M. (1987): Biochem. Biophys. Res. Commun., 144:891-900.
41. Wakil, S.J. (1958): J. Am. Chem. Soc., 80:6465-6472.
42. Wakil, S.J. and Stoops, J.K. (1983): The Enzymes, 3rd Ed.,
     vol. 16, pp. 3-42. Academic Press, New York.
43. Witters, L.A. (1981): Biochem. Biophys. Res. Commun.,
     100:872-878.
44. Witters, L.A. (1985): In: Molecular Basis of Insulin
     Action, edited by M.P. Czech, pp. 315-326. Plenum Press,
     New York.
45. Witters, L.A., Kowaloff, E.M. and Avruch, J. (1979): J.
     Biol. Chem., 254:245-247.
46. Witters, L.A., Moriarty, D. and Martin, D.B. (1979) J.
     Biol. Chem., 254:6644-6649.
47. Witters, L.A., Tipper, J.P. and Bacon, G.W. (1983): J.
     Biol. Chem., 258:5643-5648.

Insulin Action and Diabetes,
edited by H. Joseph Goren et al.
Raven Press, New York © 1988.

CURRENT ISSUES IN INSULIN ACTION

I.G. Fantus

Polypeptide Hormone Laboratory, Strathcona Medical Building,
McGill University, 3640 University Street, Room 211, Montreal,
Quebec, H3A 2B2.

INSULIN RECEPTOR PHOSPHORYLATION

The important role of autophosphorylation of the insulin receptor β-subunit and its activation as a tyrosine protein kinase has been discussed at this meeting. The first presentation in this workshop, entitled "Synthetic tyrosyl/phenylalanyl polypeptides as probes to study the characteristics of the insulin receptor protein tyrosine kinase" by D. Sahal, J. Ramachandran* and Y. Fujita-Yamaguchi (Beckman Research Institute of the City of Hope, Duarte, CA and *Genentech, Inc., South San Francisco, CA) showed that various synthetic tyrosine containing peptides are able to act as substrates and/or inhibitors of the insulin receptor enzyme. Specifically [Glu^4:Tyr^1] and [Glu^6:Ala^3:Tyr^1) are both good substrates and poor inhibitors of autophosphorylation while [Tyr^1:Ala^1:Glu^1] either ordered or random were poor substrates but potent inhibitors of both auto- and substrate phosphorylation. These polymers were also tested with the IGF-I receptor and found to have similar properties but act in general as poorer substrates. Non-tyrosine containing peptides [Phe^1:Ala^1:Glu^1] had no effects.

R. Roth, Stanford: Could you comment on the differences between the insulin and the IGF-I receptor to phosphorylate these substrates.

D. Sahal: We can use two substrates with both purified receptors and arrive at a "phosphorylation" index. This may be a useful way to characterize a mixed population of receptors.

C.R. Kahn, Boston: Have you found any peptides which serve as a better substrate for the IGF-I receptor than the insulin receptor?

D. Sahal: No.

M. Hollenberg, Calgary: In terms of characterizing differences in receptors, would anyone comment on the possible differences in insulin receptors between species in view of the kinetic differences in phosphorylation demonstrated between the rat and human receptors, or between tissues in the same species.

C.R. Kahn: If you compare the kinetics of phosphorylation of the rat and human insulin receptor, the human is much slower, and yet comparing the cDNA sequences shows that all of the phosphorylation sites, the ATP binding site and 95% of the whole sequences are homologous. A small amount of amino acid modifications outside these sites must be affecting the three dimensional folding and causing changes in the kinetics and perhaps other properties. We agree with Gary Friedenberg that the kinetics vary even in the same species as you go from tissue to tissue. I don't know if this reflects differences in receptor aggregation states or due to lipids that are extracted from the membrane with Triton, but there might be interesting information which accounts for these minor differences.

G. Friedenberg, La Jolla: Maybe I can add some more confusion to the discussion by telling you that though we see dramatic differences in the rate of autophosphorylation of receptors when isolated from cells, activation of receptors "in situ", i.e. exposure of intact cells to insulin and preservation of their phosphorylation state followed by measurement of histone kinase activity in vitro, results in identical rates of rapid activation of receptors from human and rat tissues. This suggests that the sites important for activation are phosphorylated very quickly and what we may be looking at kinetically in vitro are relatively less important sites.

J. Avruch, Boston: Based on our data I would make two general comments. One is that we have found virtually complete structural homology between phosphorylation sites when the reaction is carried out in human intact cells, rat receptors in vitro and most recently with transfected cloned human receptor given to us by Axel Ullrich. This is also congruent with the human receptor autophosphorylated in vitro and the rat receptor phosphorylated in an intact cell. From a structural point of view I don't think there are any distinctions to be made. Secondly, from a functional point of view, it is hazardous to make comparisons of activity unless done in the same experiment. In addition, comparing receptor preparations prepared at different times from different sources with different techniques may also be misleading. The kinase portion of the receptor is much more susceptible to several degrees of denaturation which are reflected in its functional properties than is the binding domain.

D. Sahal: What do you think about the fact that trypsin can activate the insulin receptor kinase?

C.R. Kahn: We have localized the sites of tryptic cleaveage in the α-subunit that are responsible for the activation. There are two sets of dibasic residues which are specifically cleaved by low concentrations of trypsin, both of which are C-terminal to the cysteine rich insulin binding site region. Both cleavages will result in receptor kinase activation and insulin-like effects. This phenomenon is analogous to the mutants described by W. Rutter in which a truncated -subunit containing receptor transfected into cells was constitutively activated.

I would agree with the preceding remarks by Dr. Avruch that the same peptide maps occur for all of the phosphorylation sites to the same extent from the human and rat insulin receptor. The kinetic differences are not explained but more confusing.

VANADATE: INSULIN-LIKE ACTION IN VIVO

Recent interest has developed in the mechanism of action of several insulinomimetic agents as an approach to elucidating the mechanism of action of insulin. In particular, vanadate, a phosphotyrosine phosphatase inhibitor, has been demonstrated to possess insulin-like effects in rat adipocytes (2,4). Furthermore, an in vivo effect to lower blood glucose concentrations in streptozotocin-diabetic rats has been demonstrated (3). The second presentation, entitled "Oral administration of vanadate normalizes blood glucose levels in streptozotocin-treated rats" by J. Meyerovitch, Z. Farfel, J. Sarb, and Y. Shechter* (5) (Sheba Medical Center and Sackler School of Medicine, Tel-Aviv and *The Weizmann Institute of Science, Rehovot, Israel) examines this effect of vanadate. High concentrations (0.8 mg/ml in the drinking water) and low concentrations (0.2 mg/ml) of vanadate lowered blood glucose levels to slightly below normal and slightly above normal from frankly hyperglycemic (400 mg/dl) levels in streptozotocin-diabetic rats after 4 days of administration with no change in insulin levels. This effect was reversible and maintained for 3 weeks with low dose treatment at which time serum vanadate concentration was 0.84 ± 0.09 ug/ml. Measurements of insulin binding and action (lipogenesis) in adipocytes demonstrated a restoration (lowering) of insulin binding to normal and of insulin sensitivity (lower ED50 for insulin) after 4 days of low dose vanadate treatment. Basal in vivo uptake of 3-0-methyl glucose by liver and muscle was enhanced in both control and diabetic rats after 4 days of high dose vanadate treatment. The animals treated with the low dose became anabolic gaining 1.25 g/day (control 3.6 g/day, untreated diabetic -1.1 g/day), while those treated with a high dose remained catabolic (-1.0 g/day). There were no hepatic or renal toxic effects noted but fluid intake decreased by about 75% even in control animals exposed to the low vanadate treatment.

J. Avruch: How much glucose was in the urine when the rats were on vanadate?

Y. Shechter, Rehovot: We didn't check. We only measured blood glucose.

J. Avruch: You may want to know since you can normalize insulin binding and sensitivity to some extent by lowering the glucose however you do it. How long have you followed them on vanadate?

Y. Shechter: Five weeks.

J. Avruch: And they continue to gain weight?

Y. Shechter: At about 1/3 the normal rate but they are certainly anabolic.

R. Whitesell, Nashville: Is it possible that the high content of 3-0-methyl glucose in the liver was the result of liver edema?

Y. Shechter: No. I don't think so.

B. Posner, Montreal: Vanadate seems to have opposite effects to insulin in a recent study in hepatocytes (1). It stimulates glycogen phosphorylase and inhibits glycogen synthase. How does this fit in with your in vivo observations?

Y. Shechter: There are two possible explanations. One is that the concentrations of vanadate which were effective in vivo, circulating concentrations of 0.8 ug/ml, fall at the low end of the dose-response curve for insulinomimetic effects in vitro, i.e. only stimulate glucose oxidation 10-15% of maximal. Other in vitro effects are mediated by higher (uM) concentrations, e.g. the toxic effect to inhibit the Na^+/K^+ ATPases. Another possibility stems from the fact that vanadate is transported into cells by the anion carrier system and is reduced to VO^{2+} (IV). This form does not appear to be an inhibitor of ATPases and so,some actions in vitro may not occur in vivo.

B. Rodrigues, Vancouver: We reported in 1985 (3) that vanadate could reverse the cardiac dysfunction in streptozotocin-diabetic rats. We have found that if given for a whole year both cardiac dysfunction is reversed and diabetic cataracts are prevented.

Y. Shechter: We reproduced the blood glucose lowering effect of vanadate initially reported by Heyliger et al but found that at the concentrations of vanadate used, five times greater than ours, the rats rapidly died. We extended the study to find nontoxic concentrations and to examine effects on adipocytes.

S. Ramanadham, Vancouver: Considering the valency state of vanadate, when we tried vanadyl sulphate we found a rise in blood glucose in less than 24h. What might be happening in less than 4 days?

Y. Shechter: In 1980 I found some insulin-like effects in adipocytes with vanadyl sulphate (6). It seems that at pH 7 to 8 vanadyl sulphate (VO^{++}) is oxidized back to vanadate (VO^{-3}) which penetrates the cell and is reduced back to Vanadyl (VO^{++}). I am not sure if VO^{++}, the most likely active agent, can enter cells directly. Perhaps it takes 4 days to build up intracellular concentrations.

J. Avruch: Insulin doesn't stimulate glucose uptake in hepatocytes but you found that vanadate did. Did you check the effect of insulin?

Y. Shechter: I do not think in vitro results correlate with in vivo since we found that insulin also increased glucose uptake in vivo. Perhaps vanadate may have effects late in the insulin action cascade. We are examining its effects in insulin resistant tissue and tissues without insulin receptors. If it is active, it may have clinical value.

K. Zierler, Baltimore: Vanadate hyperpolarizes rat skeletal muscle which I think is a very early event.

Y. Shechter: Yes.   There have been reports on increased calcium uptake by cells and hyperpolarization.

1.   Bosch, F., Arino, J., Gomez-Foix, A.M., and Guinovart, J.J. (1987): J. Biol. Chem. 262: 218-222.
2.   Dubyak, G.R., and Kleinzeller, A. (1980): J. Biol. Chem. 255: 5306-5312.
3.   Heyliger, C.E., Tahiliani, A.G., and McNeill, J.H. (1985): Science 227: 1474-1477.
4.   Kadota, S., Fantus, I.G., Hersh, B., and Posner, B.I. (1986): Biochem. Biophys. Res. Commun. 138: 174-178.
5.   Meyerovitch, J., Farfel, Z., Sack, J., and Shechter, Y. (1987): J. Biol. Chem. 262: 6658-6662.
6.   Shechter, Y., and Karlish, S.J.D. (1980): Nature: 284: 556-558.

Insulin Action and Diabetes,
edited by H. Joseph Goren et al.
Raven Press, New York © 1988.

Insulin Action In Pregnancy

Edmond A. Ryan, Louise Enns, Mary Jo O'Sullivan
and Jay S. Skyler

Department of Medicine
University of Alberta
Edmonton, Alberta
T6G 2G3
Departments of Medicine, Pediatrics and of Obstetrics and
Gynecology, University of Miami,
Miami, Florida, 33101

INTRODUCTION

Pregnancy is known to have an adverse effect on carbohydrate tolerance. Normal pregnant women display hyperinsulinemia after oral or intravenous glucose tolerance testing (9,15). Insulin has a blunted hypoglycemic response during pregnancy (6). Two to four per cent of previously normal women develop carbohydrate intolerance during pregnancy (3). Thus, pregnancy would appear to induce a state of insulin resistance. The onset of gestational diabetes and the increase in insulin requirements in diabetic pregnant women are features of the late second and the third trimester of pregnancy (3,4). The timing of these events and the rapid improvement in insulin sensitivity postpartum (8) suggests that there is a possible hormonal cause for the induction of the insulin resistance.

Many of the hormones which rise in pregnancy may have a role in producing an adverse effect on insulin action. Estradiol (E_2) and progesterone have long been associated with carbohydrate intolerance because of the hyperinsulinemia found in women taking the oral contraceptive pill (5). Cortisol and prolactin (PRL) also rise in pregnancy and may play a role. The main potential culprit is placental lactogen (PL) because of the magnitude of the rise in the level of this hormone and its similarity to growth hormone (2,13). Human chorionic gonadotropin (hCG) is the least likely to play a role in the induction of insulin resistance as the level of this hormone peaks at the end of the first trimester (16), a period at which there is no change in insulin requirements and, if anything, these requirements decrease (4).

191

We have studied insulin action during pregnancy using the euglycemic clamp technique together with oral and meal tolerance testing in vivo (14), and in vitro have used rat adipocytes to assess insulin action and how it is affected by gestational hormones.

IN VIVO STUDIES

Subjects Studied

We have studied four groups of women in our examination of insulin action during pregnancy. Group 1 were nonpregnant nondiabetic controls (NDNP). These had normal carbohydrate tolerance. Group 2 were pregnant and had normal glucose tolerance and were labeled nondiabetic pregnant (NDP). Group 3 were pregnant and had some impairment of carbohydrate tolerance when tested but did not meet the established criteria for gestational diabetes, these were called impaired glucose tolerance of pregnancy (IGTP). Finally, group 4 patients were those who had gestational diabetes (GD). The mean ages (years) $\pm$ standard error (SE) were NDNP 32.9 $\pm$ 2.1; NDP 24.8 $\pm$ 3.5; IGTP 29 $\pm$ 1.5 and GD 34.6 $\pm$ 2.6. The per cent ideal body weight for these groups was 109 $\pm$ 3.2 for NDNP; 117 $\pm$ 6.7 for NDP; 159 $\pm$ 5.8 for IGTP and 128 $\pm$ 13 for GD. The NDP group had a lower mean age than their counterparts but this did not achieve statistical significance. The patients with IGTP were more obese and this difference was significant, IGTP versus NDNP ($P<0.001$), IGTP versus NDP ($P<0.01$) but they were not significantly more obese than patients with GD. The GD patients were more obese than either NDNP or NDP but this tendency was not significant. The subjects were Caucasian, Hispanic and Black with a similar racial distribution in all groups. The study was explained in detail to all subjects each of whom gave signed informed consent in their first language.

Oral Glucose Tolerance Tests

All subjects had an oral glucose tolerance test and the results were depicted in Figure 1A. With the exception of the fasting level there was no statistical significant difference in glucose values between Group 1 (NDNP) and Group 2 (NDP). The fasting blood glucose level was lower in normal pregnancy (NDP) than nonpregnant controls NDNP ($P<0.025$). Glucose values were significantly elevated in Group 4 (GD) and Group 3 (IGTP) displayed an intermediate pattern. Insulin values were not available for most Group 4 subjects since the OGTT had been performed in the clinical laboratory just prior to recruitment for the study and it was deemed inappropriate to subject these women to a repeat glucose challenge and subsequent hyperglycemia. The insulin values, depicted in Figure 1B, clearly demonstrate that the euglycemic pregnant subjects had hyperinsulinemia and patients with IGTP could also mount a considerable insulin response. However, calculation of the incremental insulin response divided by the incremental glucose response during the first hour, Delta I/Delta G (7), gave a value of 4.01 for NDNP and 2.8 for IGTP raising the possibility of some insulin deficiency in this latter group of patients.

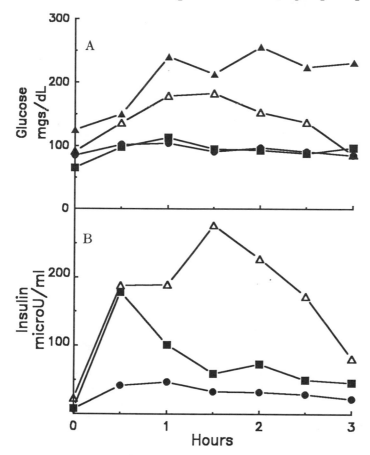

FIG. 1.   Results of Glucose Tolerance Tests

A. Glucose values are shown for Groups 1 (NDNP) (●), 2 (NDP) (■), 3 (IGTP) (△) and 4 (GD) (▲). Groups 3 and 4 displayed carbohydrate intolerance.
B. Insulin values for groups 1, 2 and 3. Group 2, despite euglycemia had hyperinsulinemia.

Meal Tolerance Testing
    The results of meal tolerance tests performed on pregnant subjects are shown in Figure 2. The meal test confirmed the abnormal tolerance test seen in Group 4 (GD) and also

demonstrated the intermediate values of Group 3 (IGTP).
Although Group 4 (GD) had a greater insulin response than Group
2 (NDP) the Delta I/Delta G ratios were 0.76 for Group 2 and
0.38 for Group 4 indicating again relative insulin deficiency
in Group 4 (GD) patients.

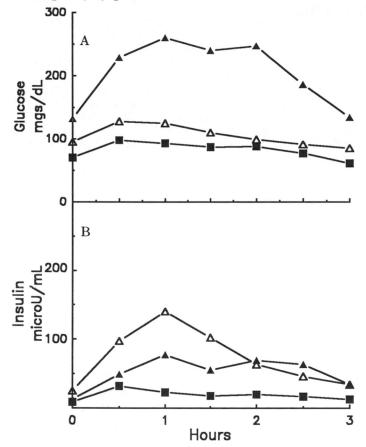

FIG. 2.   Results of Meal Tolerance Tests
A.   Glucose values are shown for Groups 2 (NDP) (■), 3(IGTP)
     (△) and 4 (GD) (▲).   Group 4 showed clear carbohydrate
     intolerance.
B.   Insulin values revealed hyperinsulinemia in Groups 3 and 4
     though the insulin increment in Group 4 is less despite
     higher glucose values.

Group 3 patients mounted a brisk insulin response and had a
Delta I/Delta G ratio of 2.07. These results confirmed that
normal pregnancy was associated with euglycemia though at the
expense of hyperinsulinemia. Patients with IGTP showed higher
insulin values and mounted an exaggerated insulin response.

Patients with GD, however, despite marked hyperglycemia showed some exaggeration of insulin response compared to NDP but this was clearly inadequate when expressed as a Delta I/Delta G ratio.

Insulin Binding Studies

The competition curves for insulin binding by erythrocytes from the four subject groups are shown in Figure 3. Essentially there was no statistical difference in the insulin binding for all four groups. IGTP tended to have slightly lower binding. Scatchard analysis (not shown) and the I_{50}'s (concentration of insulin necessary to inhibit 50% of total specific binding) were similar. The I_{50} values were 13.6 ± 3, 9.9 ± 2.1, 7.3 ± 0.9 and 10.7 ± 1.4 ng/ml for Groups 1, 2, 3, and 4 respectively. These results together with parallel Scatchard plots indicated similar binding affinities for these receptors from the different patient groups. These results demonstrated that erythrocyte insulin binding is not altered during pregnancy.

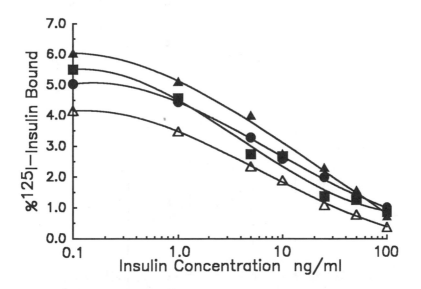

FIG. 3. Competition Curves for Insulin Binding to Erythrocytes. Symbols are as in Figures 1 and 2. Specific binding of ^{125}I insulin is shown as a function of total insulin concentration. The curves are indistinguishable, indicative of similar receptor characteristics.

Euglycemic Clamp Studies

Insulin was infused sequentially at both a low (40 $mU/M^2 \cdot min$) and high dose (240 $mU/M^2 \cdot min$) to obtain

physiological and pharmacological insulin levels. During the
low dose insulin infusion Group 1 (NDNP) subjects had a glucose
disposal rate of 213 $\pm$ 11 mg/M^2·min whilst Group 2 (NDP) had a
glucose disposal rate of 143 $\pm$ 23 mg/M^2·min (P<0.02). This
represented a 33% reduction in glucose disposal rates seen in
normal nondiabetic pregnant women compared to nonpregnant
control. Group 3 patients (IGTP) had a glucose disposal rate
of 67 $\pm$ 10 mg/M^2·min which represented a highly significant
reduction compared to NDNP (P<0.0005) and may be different from
NDP (P=0.058). Further reduction was evident in Group 4
patients (GD) whose glucose disposal rate during the low dose
insulin infusion was 57 $\pm$ 18 mg/M^2·min although this difference
was not statistically significant from Group 3 (IGTP) the
results of GD patients were significantly lower than either
NDNP or NDP. These results demonstrated that pregnant subjects
displayed a state of insulin resistance and that this
resistance is much more marked in patients with IGTP and even
further so in patients with gestational diabetes.

To further define the possible mechanism of insulin
resistance occurring in pregnancy, the high dose, 240
mU/M^2·min, insulin infusion studies were performed. During
these studies pharmacological insulin concentrations were
obtained. These results are shown in Figure 4.

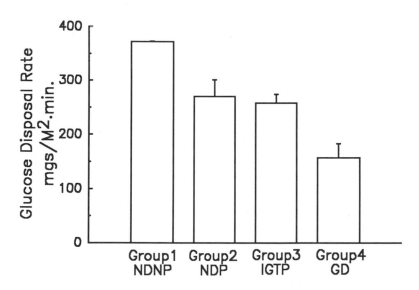

FIG. 4. Results of Euglycemic Clamp Studies During the High
Dose Insulin Infusion. Pregnancy induced a defect in insulin
action at pharmacological insulin concentrations indicative of
postbinding defect.

The glucose disposal rates for Group 1 (NDNP) subjects during the high dose insulin infusion were 372 $\pm$ 11 mg/M^2·min. In contrast, Group 2 (NDP) subjects had a 27% reduction in glucose disposal rate to 270 $\pm$ 31 mg/M^2·min (P<0.01). Group 3 (IGTP) had a slightly lower glucose disposal rate compared to Group 2 (NDP) with a rate of 258 $\pm$ 16 mg/M^2·min. This rate was not significantly different from NDP but was significantly different from NDNP (<0.0005). Gestational diabetic patients (Group 4) had markedly reduced glucose infusion rates with the high dose insulin infusion. Their glucose infusion rate was 157 $\pm$ 26 mg/M^2·min representing a 58% reduction compared to control subjects (P<0.00001). This glucose disposal rate was also significantly less than Group 2 (NDP) (P<0.025) and Group 3 (IGTP) (P<0.05). These results demonstrated that insulin resistance in pregnancy induced a decrease in maximum insulin responsivity and that this defect was aggravated when carbohydrate intolerance was present, being most severe in gestational diabetes.

Postpartum
Six subjects agreed to repeat euglycemic clamp studies in the postpartum period.

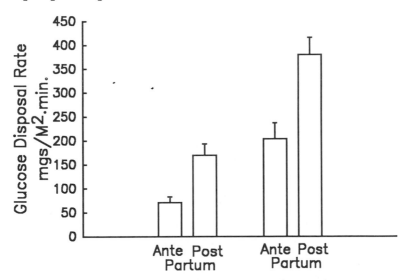

FIG. 5. Results of Euglycemic Clamp Studies in Six Subjects Antepartum and Postpartum, Low and High Dose Insulin Infusions. Two subjects each were from groups 2, 3 and 4. There was a rapid amelioration of the insulin resistance after delivery.

These included two subjects each from groups 2, 3 and 4. Four were studied within three days of delivery and one each at the fourth and ninth day postpartum. All had normal glucose tolerance tests during the postpartum period. The glucose disposal rates showed a major change as shown in Figure 5. The mean glucose disposal rate for these six patients antepartum was 71 ± 12 mg/M^2·min during the low dose insulin infusion. This increased dramatically to 170 ± 24 mg/M^2·min postpartum (P<0.005). Similar changes were seen at the high dose insulin infusion rate with an increase in the glucose disposal from 204 ± 33 to 380 ± 36 mg/M^2·min (P<0.0005). The postpartum values did not differ significantly from those obtained in the nondiabetic nonpregnant (Group 1) control subjects. This clearly demonstrated that the insulin resistance of pregnancy was ameliorated shortly after delivery. Normal glucose disposal was present postpartum regardless of the degree of transient carbohydrate intolerance antepartum.

Thus, these in vivo studies confirm the presence of insulin resistance during pregnancy and demonstrate that insulin binding is normal and that glucose disposal is reduced during infusion of pharmacological doses of insulin indicative of a postbinding defect in insulin action.

IN VITRO STUDIES

Insulin Binding and Glucose Transport
We have studied insulin action in adipocytes from pregnant and nonpregnant rats in terms of insulin receptor binding and transport of ^{14}C 3-0-methyl glucose. There was no difference in maximum insulin binding to adipocytes during pregnancy, 3.48 ± 0.5 compared to nonpregnant 3.52 ± 0.3, P=NS. However ^{14}C 3-0-methyl glucose transport was markedly reduced in adipocytes from pregnant rats 1.86 ± 0.2 versus 3.24 ± 0.4, P<0.05. The half maximum insulin concentration was similar in the glucose transport studies. These results confirmed the presence of a postbinding defect in insulin action during pregnancy.

Effects of Gestational Hormones
To examine which gestational hormones may be responsible for the induction of insulin resistance we have studied the effects of these hormones on maximum insulin binding and ^{14}C 3-0-methyl glucose transport in a primary adipocyte culture system. Using paraovarian adipocytes from virgin Sprague Dawley rats we have established a primary adipocyte culture system based on established methods (11,12) that results in the preservation of normal insulin receptor binding and ^{14}C 3-0-methyl glucose transport after three days of culture. Cell recovery was $60 \pm 3\%$ and viability (as measured by Trypan Blue exclusion of recovered cells) was in excess of 90% at 72 hours. By adding to the culture medium the hormones known to rise in pregnancy at a concentration typical of their highest level in human pregnancy, we have been able assess their effects on insulin

action. These results are summarized in Table 1.

Adding hCG or E_2 to the culture medium had no effect on maximum glucose transport 3.2 ± 0.12 and 3.12 ± 0.2 respectively versus control 3.5 ± 0.29 pmol/2x10^5 cells ·4 sec. Although hCG left maximum insulin binding unaffected, $2.73 \pm 0.52\%$ versus $2.87 \pm 0.66\%$ (control with insulin) E_2 increased maximum insulin binding to $6.5 \pm 0.5\%$ versus control (without insulin) $3.37 \pm 0.3\%$ (P<0.01).

Table 1. Effects of Gestational Hormones.

	Max. I^{125} Insulin Binding	Max. 3-0-Methyl Glucose Transport
hCG	N	N
Estradiol	↑	N
Progesterone	↓	↓
Cortisol	↓	↓
Prolactin	N	↓
hPL	N	↓

Both the cortisol and progesterone reduced maximum insulin binding and glucose transport. Maximum ^{125}I insulin binding was $0.9 \pm .3\%$ and $1.1 \pm .3\%$ for progesterone and cortisol respectively versus control $3.37 \pm 0.3\%$ (P<.001 for both). Maximum glucose transport was 1.96 ± 0.3 and 0.92 ± 0.3 pmol/2x10^5 cells ·4 sec for progesterone and cortisol respectively versus control (P<0.001). Both prolactin and hPL reduced only maximum glucose transport whilst maximum insulin binding was unchanged. Maximum glucose transport was 0.84 ± 0.25 and 1.93 ± 0.5 pmol/2x10^5 cells ·4 sec versus control (P<0.001 and P<0.005) respectively for prolactin and hPL.

These studies support the concept that gestational hormones have a role in the induction of insulin resistance of pregnancy. Cortisol and progesterone with similar effects may work through a single steroid receptor or through their own receptors which are present on adipocytes. Prolactin and placental lactogen likely exert their effects through the growth hormone receptor because of the similarity of all three hormones. The effect of growth hormone in vitro (10) is similar to what was observed in our system. The effect of estradiol in increasing insulin receptor binding has been seen in vivo (1) and is presumably counterbalanced by the negative effects on insulin binding of progesterone and cortisol. Thus as a net effect, a decrease in glucose transport is present indicative of a postbinding defect in insulin action.

These results indicate that the insulin resistance of

pregnancy, which we have shown in vivo and in vitro to be due to a postbinding defect in insulin action, is likely related to the combined effects of progesterone, cortisol, prolactin and placental lactogen.

Acknowledgement: This work was supported by funds from the Diabetes Research Institute Foundation, Miami, Florida; by the University of Miami/Southeastern Florida Regional Diabetes Program, funded by the Health Program Office, Department of Health and Rehabilitative Services, State of Florida; and by a grant from the NIH, BRSG grant no. RRO 7022-149 (Dr. O'Sullivan); by an Establishment grant from the Alberta Heritage Foundation for Medical Research and by a grant from the Central Research Fund of the University of Alberta.

References
1. Ballejo, G., Saleem, T.H., Khan-Dawood, F.S., Tsibris, J.C.M. and Spellacy W.N. (1983) The effect of sex steroids on insulin binding by target tissues in the rat. Contraception, 28: 413-21.
2. Genazzani, A.R., Cocola, F., Neri, P. and Fioretti, P. (1972): Human chorionic somatomammotropin (HCS) plasma levels in normal and pathological pregnancies and their correlation with the placental function. Acta Endocrinol, 71, Supp 167: 5-39.
3. Hadden, D.R. (1980): Screening for abnormalities of carbohydrate metabolism in pregnancy 1966- 1977: the Belfast Experience. Diabetes Care, 3:440-6.
4. Jovanovic, L., Druzin, M. and Peterson, C.M. (1981): Effect of euglycemia on the outcome of pregnancy in insulin-dependent diabetic women as compared with normal control subjects. Am J Med, 71: 921-7.
5. Kalkhoff, R.K. (1980): Relative sensitivity of postpartum gestational diabetic women to oral contraceptive agents and other metabolic stress. Diabetes Care, 3: 421-4.
6. Knopp, R.H., Ruder, H.J., Herrera, E. and Freinkel, N. (1970): Carbohydrate metabolism in pregnancy. VII. Insulin tolerance during late pregnancy in the fed and fasted rat. Acta Endocrinol, 65: 352-60.
7. Kuhl, C. and Holst, J.J. (1976): Plasma glucagon and the insulin:glucagon ratio in gestational diabetes. Diabetes, 25: 16-23
8. Lawrence, R.D. and Oakley, W. (1942): Pregnancy and diabetes. Quart J Med, 11: 45-75.
9. Lind, T., Billewicz, W.Z. and Brown, G. (1973): A serial study of changes occurring in the oral glucose tolerance test during pregnancy. J Obstet Gynaec Brit Commonw, 80: 1033-9.
10. Maloff, B.L., Levine, J.H. and Lockwood, D.H. (1980): Direct effects of growth hormone on insulin action in rat adipose tissue maintained in vitro. Endocrinol., 107: 538-

44
11. Marshall, S. : Kinetics of insulin receptor biosynthesis and membrane insertion: relationship to cellular function. Diabetes, 32: 319–25.
12. Marshall, S., Garvey, W.T. and Geller, M. (1984): Primary culture of isolated adipocytes: a new model to study insulin receptor regulation and insulin action. J Biol Chem, 259: 6376–84.
13. Niall, H.D., Hogan, M.L. and Sauer, R. (1971): Sequences of pituitary and placental lactogenic and growth hormones: Evolution from a primordial peptide by gene reduplication. Proc Natl Acad Sci USA, 68: 866–9.
14. Ryan, E.A., O'Sullivan, M.J. and Skyler, J.S. (1985): Insulin action during pregnancy: studies with the euglycemic clamp technique. Diabetes, 34: 380–389.
15. Spellacy, W.N. and Goetz, F.C.(1963): Plasma insulin in normal late pregnancy. N Engl J Med, 268: 988–91.
16. Teoh, E.S. (1967): Chorionic gonadotrophin in the serum and urine of Asian women in normal pregnancy. J Obstet Gynaecol Br Commonw, 74: 74–9.

Insulin Action and Diabetes,
edited by H. Joseph Goren et al.
Raven Press, New York © 1988.

IMPAIRED PROTEIN KINASE C ACTIVITY IN

INSULIN-RESISTANT TISSUES OF

GENETICALLY OBESE (fa/fa) RATS

Gerald van de Werve

Laboratoire d'Endocrinologie Metabolique,
Departement de Nutrition,
Universite de Montreal, Quebec

Activation of calcium- and phospholipid- dependent protein kinase (PKC) (1) by phorbol esters causes insulin-like effects. These include phosphorylation of the subunit of the insulin receptor and activation of tyrosine aminotransferase in hepatoma cells (2), stimulation of lipogenesis in adipocytes (3) and of glucose transport in heart (4). In the presence of insulin, however, phorbol esters counteract insulin action (2-4). Since PKC thus modulates insulin action, a possible defect of this kinase could be associated with insulin resistance. This hypothesis was tested in tissues (heart and liver) of genetically obese (fa/fa) rats that are resistant to insulin (5).

In isolated perfused hearts from lean rats, phorbol myristate acetate (PMA) or insulin caused each a dose-dependent increase in glucose transport, which was unaffected by the concomittent addition of the Ca^{++} inophore A23187 (2uM). Maximal stimulation was about fourfold for the phorbol ester and tenfold for the hormone.

In hearts from obese animals, glucose transport was insensitive to PMA and the maximal stimulation by insulin was reduced by 50%. When A23187 was added in combination with PMA, the ionophore then allowed a stimulatory effect of PMA to occur, of similar magnitude to that seen in lean rat heart. When the inophore was infused together with insulin, the maximal response to the hormone was partially restored.

When an optimal dose (200 ng/ml) of PMA was combined with increasing insulin concentrations, the dose-response curve for glucose transport in lean rat heart was shifted to the right (by more than one order of magnitude) but the maximal response was not affected. In contrast, PMA did not change the insulin-sensitivity of glucose transport in hearts from obese animals.

In an attempt to down-regulate PKC in vivo, lean rats were treated intraperitoneally with PMA (50 ug/kg) body wt. for two days). The hearts were then isolated and perfused with PMA or insulin in vitro. The treatment in vivo resulted in a loss of responsiveness of glucose transport to PMA and induced a resistance to insulin comparable to the one prevailing in the untreated obese rat heart.

PKC activity was directly measured in extracts of soluble and particulate fractions of hearts purified on DEAE cellulose. Treatment of perfused hearts from both groups of animals with PMA (200 ng/ml) provoked a decrease in PKC activity in the soluble fraction. A complementary increase in PKC activity in the particulate fraction was however only observed in tissue preparations from lean rats.

As liver from fa/fa rats was shown to be insulin-resistant in vivo (see ref. 5), the inactivation of glycogen synthase by PMA- or vasopressin-stimulated PKC was studied in isolated hepatocytes. A dose-dependent inactivation of glycogen synthase by PMA or vasopressin was observed in hepatocytes isolated from lean but not from obese animals.

The present results indicated impaired PKC in insulin-resistant tissues of the fa/fa rat. The nature of the defect is unknown but might be related to reduced sensitivity of the kinase to Ca^{++} because phorbol esters did stimulate glucose transport in obese rat heart provided that $[Ca^{++}]$ was increased at the same time by the ionophore A23187. Furthermore, the anchoring of PKC to the plasma membrane is calcium-dependent (6) and translocation of this enzyme from cytosol to membranes is impaired in obese rat heart. The latter observation is consistent with a role of the membrane-bound PKC in PMA stimulation of glucose transport in heart.

A link between PKC defect and insulin resistance is suggested by the following observations: (i) impaired stimulation of glucose transport in obese rat heart by PMA and insulin; (ii) restoration of PMA-stimulated transport and partial reversal of insulin resistance by calcium mobilization; (iii) induction of PMA-unresponsiveness and insulin resistance of glucose transport in hearts from lean animals pretreated with PMA in vivo; (iv) impaired inactivation by PMA and vasopressin of glycogen synthase in hepatocytes from obese rats.

Although PKC activation does not seem to be an obligatory step in insulin action (7-10) part of the insulin resistance involves a defective PKC because this enzyme modulates insulin action.

PKC and the insulin receptor kinase might indeed share common substrates explaining how similar biological responses are elicited both by insulin and by agents which stimulate PKC. Competitive phosphorylation of these substrates by both kinases might explain antagonistic effects of PKC activation on insulin action. It remains to be defined under which physiological conditions such interactions between insulin action and PKC take place.

ACKNOWLEDGEMENTS

Our work performed at the Laboratories de Recherches Metaboliques, University of Geneva (Switzerland), has been supported by grant no. 3.822.086 from the National Swiss Science Foundation (Berne, Switzerland) and by a grant-in-aid from Nestle S.A. (Vevey, Switzerland).

REFERENCES

(1) Nishizuka, Y (1984) Nature 308: 693-698

(2) Takayama, S, White, MF, Lauris, V and Kahn, RC (1984) Proc Nat Acad Sci USA 81: 7797-7801

(3) van de Werve, G, Proietto, J and Jeanrenaud, B (1985) Biochem J 225: 523-527

(4) van de Werve, G, Zaninetti, D, Lang, U, Vallotton, MB and Jeanrenaud, B (1987) Diabetes 36: 310-314.

(5) Jeanrenaud, B, Halimi, S, and van de Werve, G (1985) Diab Metab Rev 1: 261-291

(6) Wolf, M, LeVine III, H, May Jr, WS, Cuatrecasas, P and Sahyoun, H (1985) Nature 317: 546-549.

(7) Blackshear, PJ, Witters, LA, Girard, PR, Kuo, JF and Quamo, SN (1985) J Biol Chem 260: 13304-13315

(8) Jacobs, S and Cuatrecasas, P (1986) J Biol Chem 261: 934-939

(9) Glynn, BP, Colliton, JW, McDermott, JM and Witters, LA (1986) Biochem Biophys Res Commun 135: 1119-1125

(10) Klip, A and Ramlal, T (1987) Biochem J 242: 131-136

Insulin Action and Diabetes,
edited by H. Joseph Goren et al.
Raven Press, New York © 1988.

SYNDROMES OF INSULIN RESISTANCE: PATHOGENIC MECHANISMS

Phillip Gorden, Richard Arakaki, Dominique Rouiller,
Richard Comi, Elaine Collier and Simeon I. Taylor

Diabetes Branch, National Institute of Diabetes and
Digestive and Kidney Diseases, National Institutes
of Health, Bethesda, Maryland 20892

INTRODUCTION

The regulation of blood glucose and other metabolic
processes can be looked upon schematically as a closed system
whereby insulin is secreted from the β cell of the islets of
Langerhans, transported in plasma, and recognized by target
cells that transduce a regulatory group of signals (Fig. 1).
Viewed in this way, it is clear that impairment of insulin
action can occur at many levels but defects at the level of
the target cell are the most frequent. Since the insulin
receptor is the initial site of insulin action at the cellular
level, it has become a focal point in the study of insulin
resistance.
Insulin action is a function of the insulin-receptor
complex on the plasma membrane of the target cell. Insulin
itself may be quantitatively or qualitatively deficient and
likewise the insulin receptor may be quantitatively or
qualitatively deficient. In the present discussion we will
focus on the quantitative and qualitative aspects of the
insulin receptor and its role in the pathogenesis of insulin
resistance in clinical disease states.

Biogenesis and Degradation of the Insulin Receptor

The insulin receptor is an integral membrane glycoprotein
of most cells. The receptor exists in the plasma membrane
predominantly as a disulfide-linked heterodimer consisting of
2 alpha subunits and 2 beta subunits (Fig. 2). The α subunit
is external to the membrane, whereas the β subunit is a
transmembrane protein. The α subunit contains the insulin
binding domain, and the β subunit is the tyrosine specific
protein kinase that undergoes autophosphorylation.

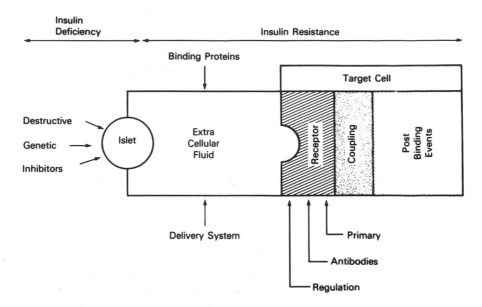

FIG. 1.   Mechanisms of insulin deficiency and resistance.

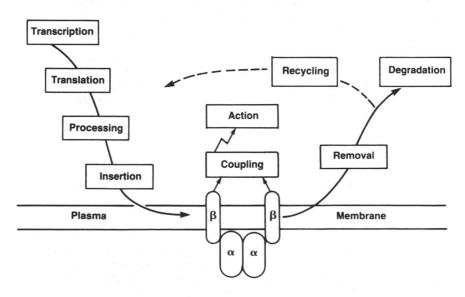

FIG. 2.   Regulation of cell surface insulin receptor
          concentration.

The receptor is encoded by a single gene and synthesized as
a single chain prorecepter which undergoes a number of
processing steps; these include N-linked glycosylation with
transition of the high-mannose type to complex type chains,
enzymatic cleavage, and fatty acylation (Fig. 3) (9)(14)
(24)(26)(38)(44).

Like other membrane receptor proteins, the ligand bound
complex can be internalized by the cell through an endocytotic
mechanism (19). The internalized ligand and receptor may then
be degraded or recycled to the plasma membrane as a complex or
become dissociated in the acidic environment of the endosome
and be processed independently of each other (Fig. 2)(19).

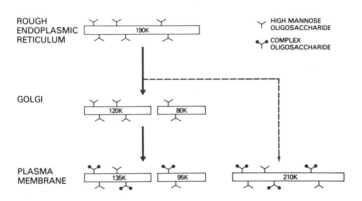

FIG. 3. Schematic representation of insulin receptor
         biogenesis.

Pathology of Receptor Regulation

High concentrations of insulin in vitro and hyperinsulinemia in vivo lead to a state of insulin receptor "down
regulation" (3)(18). Under these circumstances binding sites
are lost from the cell surface presumably by the process of
receptor mediated endocytosis (19). Regardless of whether
hyperinsulinemia is primary or secondary to a cellular defect
in insulin action, the loss of cell surface binding further
impairs insulin response. Recently, the converse of ligand-
induced receptor depletion has been demonstrated; under
circumstances of impoverished insulin secretion, endocytosis
is impaired and cell surface receptors are conserved (5).

In general, insulin resistant states such as obesity, type
II diabetes, and lipoatrophic diabetes are associated with a
reversible state of receptor "down regulation" (23).
Recently, in type II diabetes loss of the α-β coupling
function of the insulin receptor has been demonstrated (Fig.
4)(4)(7)(16). This appears to be relatively specific for the
insulin receptor since the IGF-I receptors on the same cells
are unaffected (7). The mechanism that produces a decrease in
tyrosine phosphorylation (i.e., β subunit function) relative
to insulin binding (i.e., α subunit function) is unknown, but
to the extent that the β subunit subserves a transduction role
in insulin signaling, this defect is a potential molecular
site of insulin resistance. Further, this defect, like the
down regulation process itself, appears to be reversible with
therapy (17).

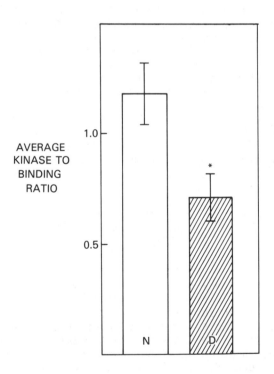

FIG. 4. Comparison of the ratio of insulin-stimulated
tyrosine kinase to insulin binding activities of lectin
purified red cell insulin receptors from normal (N) and
type II diabetic (D) subjects (* = $p < 0.05$).

Clinical Phenotypes of Receptor Diseases

A variety of insulin resistant syndromes have been described based on clinical features and insulin receptor α and β subunit function (23)(27)(43). Since in all of these syndromes the evidence linking the clinical phenotype to the mechanism of insulin resistance remain undiscovered, we will first describe the syndromes and then separately discuss the nature of the receptor defects that have been elucidated. Table 1 lists the clinical phenotypes and some of their distinguishing characteristics. There are several features that are frequently present. These include extreme insulin resistance, hyperinsulinemia, and either euglycemia or hyperglycemia. The blood glucose concentration is a function of the circulating insulin concentration rather than the degree of insulin resistance. Even in extreme insulin resistance blood glucose may be normal with the presence of marked hyperinsulinemia. Acanthosis nigricans is frequently present and in premenopausal women polycystic ovaries, hirsutism, androgen excess and virilization are common.

The type B form of insulin resistance is an autoimmune syndrome characterized by autoantibody production to the insulin receptor (Table 1). This may result in a metabolic state of hyperglycemia, hypoglycemia or alternating hyperglycemia and hypoglycemia. This abnormality results from the binding of the autoantibody to the insulin receptor; the receptor per se appears to be normal and in fact functions normally when the autoantibody disappears. This is representative of a general class of autoimmune endocrine and neurotransmitter disorders such as Graves' disease and myasthenia gravis (8)(27)(41).

Mechanisms Involved with Primary Receptor Diseases: Accelerated Receptor Degradation and Biosynthetic Abnormalities

The understanding of the mechanisms of receptor defects is at a very preliminary stage, and as previously mentioned the molecular defect in receptor function bears no particular relationship to the clinical phenotype.

It is now possible to measure separately α subunit and β subunit function, and characterize their general properties. Furthermore, the cloning of the cDNA for the insulin receptor has not only provided molecular probes but has permitted the elucidation of the amino acid sequence of the proreceptor. These developments plus biosynthetic and other labeling techniques have provided the concepts and tools to probe the molecular pathology of the receptor.

TABLE 1.   Insulin Receptor Related Syndromes of Extreme
                    Insulin Resistance[a]

Syndrome	Special clinical features	Insulin binding and reference
Leprechaunism	Intra-uterine growth retardation and fasting hypoglycemia	Normal or decreased (40, 42)
Type A	Normal weight[b]	Normal or decreased (23,27,43)
Rabson Mendenhall	Dystrophic nails and teeth ? Pineal hyperplasia	Decreased (33)
Type B	Antireceptor antibodies and other autoimmune manifestations	Decreased (8,27,41)

[a]All these syndromes are typically associated with acanthosis nigricans, polycystic ovaries, and hirsutism.
[b]Usually seen in young females, but occasionally in males. When these phenotypic features are seen in the presence of obesity, the receptor abnormality, if any, is usually "down regulation."

Since the steady state receptor concentration is a function of synthesis and removal (Fig. 2), it is first necessary to determine which limb of the process is affected. Down regulation is the accelerated removal of the ligand bound receptor by receptor mediated endocytosis. It is possible, however, that either this or some other mechanism could lead to accelerated receptor degradation. When cell surface receptors from a number of patients with extreme insulin resistance were labeled by the Na ^{125}I/lactoperoxidase method and turnover rates determined, there was only a modest increase in receptor degradation rate (i.e., $\sim$ 40%) regardless of whether cells contained normal or severely reduced receptor concentration. Thus, it appears that an accelerated degradation rate is not a major mechanism accounting for very low cell surface receptor concentration (32). Therefore, the major focus of study has been on the biosynthetic process.

Though the cDNA for the insulin receptor gene has been cloned, the structure of the insulin receptor gene has not been published and very little is known about the regulation of this gene. Thus far no cDNA for a mutant insulin receptor has been described (11), but there are preliminary data using linkage analysis to suggest that mutant genes will be found (1)(29).

Several defects at the molecular level have been identified in insulin resistant states (Table 2). (a) Thus far the earliest defect in the biosynthetic pathway to be clearly distinguished is at the level of mRNA where Northern blot analysis has shown a marked decrease in total insulin receptor mRNA (36). This finding probably accounts for the quantitative deficiency in proreceptor and mature subunits. In normal cells, insulin receptor mRNAs of different sizes (lengths) are produced, however, no preferential loss of a particular length is identified in abnormal cells. The mechanism underlying the deficient total message is unknown. (b) In a different pattern, normal amounts of mRNA, proreceptor, and mature subunits are produced as demonstrated by Northern blot analysis (36), and biosynthetic labeling (25)(33). The mature receptor, however, is not inserted into the plasma membrane. It is presumed that the intracellular receptor is either degraded or otherwise prevented from becoming inserted into the plasma membrane. (c) The aforementioned defects represent situations where α and β subunits are concomitantly reduced. In general, the most common situation observed is the reduction of function in both subunits (23). However, a defect has been described where α subunit function is normal in multiple cell types but β subunit function is markedly reduced (20)(21). That is, tyrosine kinase activity is absent, but insulin binding is normal. Thus far in this situation no inhibitor of phosphorylation has been identified. Paradoxically in this patient while β subunit function is markedly reduced in erythrocytes, monocytes and fibroblasts, this function is normal in E.B. virus transformed lymphocytes (22). (d) All of the above situations refer to quantitative reductions in α subunit function, β subunit function or both. A defect, however, has been described where these functions are essentially normal but where α subunit function is qualitatively abnormal with respect to dissociation characteristics, temperature and pH regulation of insulin binding (40)(42).

TABLE 2. Loci of Molecular Defect in Human Insulin Receptor

Level of Biosyn- thetic Defect	Method of Detection	Reference
DNA	Southern blot analysis with RFLP probes	(1)(11) (29)
mRNA	Northern blot analysis	(36)
Proreceptor	Biosynthetic labeling	(25)(33)
β subunit	Tyrosine phosphory- lation	(20)(21)
Mature cell surface α and β subunits	Equilibrium binding and covalent cross- linking	(40)(42)

Abnormal Processing of the Insulin Receptor:
Potential Model for Disease States

Since the insulin receptor undergoes a complex series of
processing events, abnormalities could potentially exist at
any level. None, however, have been described in human
cells. In Chinese hamster ovary cells (CHO), two different
types of mutations in glycosylation have been described that
result in altered insulin receptor function (37). The first
is the transfer of a shortened high-mannose form from
dolichol-pyrophosphate to the asparagine of the nascent
polypeptide (i.e., Man_5 for Man_9). The truncated high-mannose
form is further processed to complex oligosaccharide with the
resultant mature receptor having a markedly increased
affinity. It otherwise functions normally. The second mutant
cell line lacks the enzyme N-acetylglucosaminyl transferase I
which is necessary for processing high-mannose forms to
complex type oligosaccharides. This results in a major
decrease in insulin receptor affinity. In both cases the
defect is specific for the insulin receptor. The IGF-I
receptor on these cells is unaffected. Since carbohydrate
changes generally result in altered metabolism and/or
transport of the receptor, it is unclear why these defects
lead to altered receptor function.
    Another way to study abnormalities in glycosylation is by
the use of inhibitors of enzymatic cleavage or of transferase
function. Recently glucosidase inhibitors have been used to

block glucose removal from the core oligosaccharide (2). Under these conditions insulin binding is reduced due to a quantitative reduction in cell surface receptors, but the receptors present in the plasma membrane appear to be qualitatively normal. This has led to the concept that glucose removal from the core oligosaccharide is an important signal for insulin receptor movement from one cellular compartment to another. Whether these effects are due to alteration in the physical properties of the glycoprotein or to some other mechanism is presently unknown.

Future Studies: Transcriptional and Translational Mechanisms

Site specific mutagenesis has recently been employed to study receptor function (6)(10)(12). A number of recombinant mutants have been produced to probe single amino acid substitutions at critical points in the α and β subunit. These studies have great promise for elucidating the normal mechanisms of signal transduction and their abberations. Recently, monoclonal antibodies to specific regions of the α and β subunits have been employed to similarly probe the mechanisms of receptor function (15)(34)(35).

While glycosylation and proteolytic cleavage are the major post-translational modifications described for the insulin receptor, other processing steps have begun to be elucidated. One of the most recently described is fatty acylation, where both myristic and palmitic acids are found covalently linked to the mature insulin receptor. The α subunit contains only amide-linked fatty acids while the β subunit contains fatty acids in both amide and ester linkages (26). While the function of fatty acylation of the insulin receptor is unknown, it has been found that myristylation is a critical feature of the p^{60} src transforming protein of Rous sarcoma virus (28).

Glucocorticoid will induce the insulin receptor and this effect can be seen at the level of the proreceptor (13)(39). The increased proreceptor synthesis induced by glucocorticoid is accompanied by an increase in receptor mRNA (30)(31) (Rouiller, D. et al., manuscript in preparation). Whether this is due to increased transcription of the gene is still under study, but this represents at least the first steps in understanding the regulation of the insulin receptor gene.

References

1. Accili, D., Elbein, S., McKeon, C., and Taylor, S. I. (1987): Diabetes, 36(1):21A.

2. Arakaki, R. F., Hedo, J. A., Collier, E., and Gorden, P. (1987): J. Biol. Chem., 262(24):11886-11892.
3. Bar, R. S., Gorden, P., Roth, J., Kahn, C. R., and DeMeyts, P. (1976): J. Clin. Invest., 58:1123-1135.
4. Caro, J. F., Ittoop, O., Pories, W. J., Meelheim, D., Flickinger, E. G., Thomas, F., Jenquin, M., Silverman, J. F., Khazanie, P. G., and Sinha, M. K. (1986): J. Clin. Invest., 78:249-258.
5. Carpentier, J.-L., Robert, A., Grunberger, G., Van Obberghen, E., Freychet, P., Orci, L., and Gorden, P. (1986): J. Clin. Endocrinol. Metab., 63:151-155.
6. Chou, C. K., Dull, T. J., Russell, D. S., Gherzi, R., Lebwohl, D., Ullrich, A., and Rosen, O. M. (1987): J. Biol. Chem., 262:1842-1847.
7. Comi, R. J., Grunberger, G., and Gorden, P. (1987): J. Clin. Invest., 79:453-462.
8. Dons, R. F., Havlik, R., Taylor, S. I., Baird, K. L., Chernick, S. S., and Gorden, P. (1983): J. Clin. Invest., 72:1072-1080.
9. Ebina, Y., Ellis, L., Jarnagin, K., Edery, M., Graf, L., Clauser, E., Ou, J., Masiarz, F., Kan, Y. W., Goldfine, I. D., Roth, R. A., and Rutter, W. J. (1985): Cell, 40:747-758.
10. Ebina, Y., Araki, E., Taira, M., Shimada, F., Mori, M., Craik, C. S., Siddle, K., Pierce, S. B., Roth, R. A., and Rutter, W. J. (1987): Proc. Natl. Acad. Sci., USA, 84:704-708.
11. Elbein, S. C., Corsetti, L., Ullrich, A., and Permutt, M. A. (1986): Proc. Natl. Acad. Sci., USA, 83:5223-5227.
12. Ellis, L., Clauser, E., Morgan, D. O., Edery, M., Roth, R. A., and Rutter, W. J. (1986): Cell, 45:721-732.
13. Fantus, I. G., Saviolakis, G. A., Hedo, J. A., and Gorden, P. (1982): J. Biol. Chem., 257:8277-8283.
14. Forsayeth, J., Maddux, B., and Goldfine, I. D. (1986): Diabetes, 35:837-846.
15. Forsayeth, J. R., Caro, J. F., Sinha, M. K., Maddux, B. A., and Goldfine, I. D. (1987): Proc. Natl. Acad. Sci., USA, 84:3448-3451.
16. Freidenberg, G. R., Henry, R. R., Klein, H. H., Reichart, D. R., and Olefsky, J. M. (1987): J. Clin. Invest., 79:240-250.
17. Freidenberg, G., Reichart, D., and Henry, R. (1987): Diabetes, 36(1):157A.
18. Gavin, J. R., III, Roth, J., Neville, D. M., Jr., DeMeyts, P., and Buell, D. N. (1974): Proc. Natl. Acad. Sci., USA, 71:84-88.
19. Gorden, P., Carpentier, J.-L., and Orci, L. (1985): In: Diabetes/Metabolism Reviews, edited by R. A. DeFronzo, pp. 99-117, John Wiley & Sons, Inc., New York.

20. Grigorescu, F., Flier, J. S., and Kahn, C. R. (1984):
    J. Biol. Chem., 259:15003-15006.
21. Grunberger, G., Zick, Y., and Gorden, P. (1984):
    Science, 223:932-934.
22. Grunberger, G., McElduff, A., Comi, R. J., Podskalny,
    J. M., Taylor, S. I., and Gorden, P. (1985): Clin.
    Res. 33:614A.
23. Grunberger, G., and Gorden, P. (1986): In: Clinical
    Diabetes Mellitus: A Problem-Oriented Approach,
    edited by J. K. Davidson, pp.77-88, Thieme-Stratton,
    Inc., New York.
24. Hedo, J. A., and Gorden, P. (1985): Horm. Metabol.
    Res., 17:487-490.
25. Hedo, J. A., Moncada, V. Y., and Taylor, S. I. (1985):
    J. Clin. Invest., 76:2355-2361.
26. Hedo, J. A., Collier, E., and Watkinson, A. (1987):
    J. Biol. Chem., 262:954-957.
27. Kahn, C. R., Flier, J. S., Bar, R. S., Archer, J. A.,
    Gorden, P., Martin, M. M., and Roth, J. (1976): New
    Engl. J. Med., 294:739-745.
28. Kamps, M. P., Buss, J. E., and Sefton, B. M. (1986):
    Cell, 45:105-112.
29. Kriauciunas, K., Mueller-Wieland, D., Kahn, C. R., and
    Taub, R. (1986): Diabetes 35(1):1A.
30. McDonald, A. R., Maddux, B. A., Okabayashi, Y., Wong,
    K. Y., Hawley, D. M., and Goldfine, I. D. (1987):
    Diabetes, 36(6):779-781.
31. McDonald, A. R., Maddux, B. A., and Goldfine, I. D.
    (1987): Diabetes, 36(1):8A.
32. McElduff, A., Hedo, J. A., Taylor, S. I., Roth, J., and
    Gorden, P. (1984): J. Clin. Invest., 74:1366-1374.
33. Moncada, V. Y., Hedo, J. A., Serrano-Rios, M., and
    Taylor, S. I. (1986): Diabetes, 35:802-807.
34. Morgan, D. O., Ho, L., Korn, L. J., and Roth, R. A.
    (1986): Proc. Natl. Acad. Sci., USA, 83:328-332.
35. Morgan, D. O., and Roth, R. A. (1987): Proc. Natl.
    Acad. Sci., USA, 84:41-45.
36. Ojamaa, K., Hedo, J. A., Roberts, C. T., Jr., Gorden,
    P., Ullrich, A., and Taylor, S. I. (1987): Amer.
    Diabetes Asso. Annual Mtg. Abs., p. 1A.
37. Podskalny, J. M., Rouiller, D. G., Grunberger, G.,
    Baxter, R. C., McElduff, A., and Gorden, P. (1986):
    J. Biol. Chem., 261:14076-14081.
38. Ronnett, G. V., Knutson, V. P., Kohanski, R. A.,
    Simpson, T. L., and Lane, M. D. (1984): J. Biol.
    Chem., 259:4566-4575.
39. Rouiller, D. G., McElduff, A., Hedo, J. A., and Gorden,
    P. (1985): J. Clin. Invest., 76:645-649.

40. Taylor, S. I., Roth, J., Blizzard, R. M., and Elders, M. J. (1981): Proc. Natl. Acad. Sci., USA, 78: 7157-7161.
41. Taylor, S. I., Grunberger, G., Marcus-Samuels, B., Underhill, L. H., Dons, R. F., Ryan, J., Roddam, R. F., Rupe, C. E., and Gorden, P. (1982): N. Engl. J. Med., 307:1422-1426.
42. Taylor, S. I., and Leventhal, S. (1983): J. Clin. Invest., 71:1676-1685.
43. Taylor, S. I. (1985): In: Diabetes/Metabolism Reviews, edited by R. A. DeFronzo, pp. 171-202, John Wiley & Sons, Inc., New York.
44. Ullrich, A., Bell, J. R., Chen, E. Y., Herrera, R., Petruzzelli, L. M., Dull, T. J., Gray, A., Coussens, L. Liao, Y.-C., Tsubokawa, M., Mason, A., Seeburg, P. H., Grunfeld, C., Rosen, O. M., and Ramachandran, J. (1985): Nature, 313:756-761.

Acknowledgment: We wish to thank Mrs. Carla Hendricks and Mrs. Mary Rushing for their assistance in the preparation of this manuscript.

Insulin Action and Diabetes,
edited by H. Joseph Goren et al.
Raven Press, New York © 1988.

HYPOTHESIS REGARDING THE DEFECT IN INSULIN ACTION
IN OBESITY FROM MODELING OF CLINICAL DATA

Richard N. Bergman

Department of Physiology and Biophysics
USC Medical School, Los Angeles, CA 90003

One fundamental rationale for the study of insulin action is to understand its implications for the pathogenesis of various metabolic conditions, such as obesity, aging and endocrine disorders including diabetes mellitus. Thus, it is a laudable goal to try to investigate the specific cellular-level defects which are manifest as insulin resistance in the intact individual. One profitable approach has been the study of isolated tissues harvested from animal models of disease, or even from human patients. However, as the animal models usually can be differentiated from the human condition, and the specific tissues of interest (for example, muscle cells) may not be readily available for collection, another approach may be needed.

Jerrold Olefsky and his colleagues at the University of California at San Diego have for some years been examining the quantitative relationship between plasma insulin and insulin action in vivo. The actions of insulin studied are the increase in the rate of glucose utilization (R_d), and suppression of the endogenous rate of glucose production (R_a). In collaboration with Olefsky and Dr. Rudy Prager we have utilized computer modeling to analyze the time dependent effects of insulin on R_d during glucose clamp experiments. In these experiments, insulin is infused rapidly elevating the plasma insulin level, and R_d increases slowly, achieving a new elevated steady-state ($R_d$ss) by 3 hours, which is a reflection of the insulin sensitivity of the individual. Prager et al. have carefully examined the time courses of the R_d responses to various insulin doses, in normal weight and obese subjects.

The clear differences in dynamics between normal-weight and obese subjects are described in reference 1; they can be summarized as follows: In all subjects, as insulin dose was increased the rate of attainment of $R_d$ss was increased, while the rate of descent was slower. Also, at equivalent insulin doses, $R_d$ss was achieved more slowly and deactivated more rapidly in obese than normal weight subjects.

We felt that these provocative, if nonlinear differences in R_d dynamics between normal-weight and obese subjects might yield clues as to the cellular-level defect which was responsible for insulin resistance in the obese. Expressed as the insulin sensitivity index, S_I (2), obese subjects had S_I reduced by 2/3 from normal. To interpret the dynamic results we proposed a quantitative model of insulin action at the level of the cell (Figure 1). The model "cell" represents the individual roles of insulin and glucose itself in determining glucose utilization by all the body's tissues. Thus, on the surface of the stereotypical cell are transporters (T_0) which carry glucose into the cell in the absence of insulin; other insulin-dependent transporters shuttle from the cell interior (T_i) to the membrane (T_m). Insulin is presumed to enter the interstitial space, bind to the cell surface receptors and generate putative signal "X(t)"; the latter either degrades or increases the transfer rate of transporters to the surface of the cell. Rate of glucose uptake by the "cell" was deemed proportional to the number of cell-associated transporters as well as the ambient (interstitial) glucose level. Of course, it is understood although the activation of transporters in this model is represented by physical translocation to the membrane locus, this could also represent chemical activation of the transport unit, as well as physical relocation to the membrane site.

This model accounted for the R_d dynamics discussed above for the patients. In accounting for the data, parameters were calculated which represented the transduction of the plasma insulin "signal" into the cell (k_2), the degradation rate of the mediator signal (k_3) as well as the fractional rate of re-internalization of membrane-associated transporter molecules (k_1).

Parameter values obtained from the normal versus the obese data leads to a specific hypothesis of the mechanism of insulin resistance in the obese subjects. From the modeling process, in the obese subjects the total number of transport units was reduced 29%. However, this reduction could not account for the 2/3 reduction in insulin sensitivity of the obese. In addition, less transport units could not, by itself explain the dynamic changes in the patterns of increase and decrease in R_d during clamps. The most significant contribution to insulin resistance was a 5-fold increase in parameter k_1 in the obese subjects compared to controls. This highly significant difference indicates that the membrane-associated (or activated) glucose transporters were much more stable in normal individuals -- the mean residence time on the membrane for transporters in normal individuals is 45 minutes, *but this time is reduced to just 9 minutes in the obese*, according to the simulation.

The modeling study described, therefore, leads to a very specific hypothesis of the insulin resistance of obesity, to whit, that *the insulin resistance of obesity is primarily due to an instability of activated (possibly membrane-bound) trans-porters*, such that the average time spent by a typical transporter in the active state is reduced from 45 to just 6 minutes. This single hypothesis can explain most of the decrease in $R_q$ss in the obese, as well as the profound dynamic contrasts between the normal and obese individuals.

Of course a modeling study of this type cannot provide absolute proof for or against any specific cellular hypothesis of insulin resistance. The latter requires direct studies of the kinetics of movement (activation/deactivation) of glucose transporters in skeletal muscle cells--those cells responsible for the insulin resistance of obesity. Nevertheless this study can serve to pinpoint a direction for future studies at the cellular and organelle level. It emphasizes that we must observe not just the number of transport units and their distribution between cellular and intracellular loci (or between activated versus deactivated states), but we must focus on the *kinetics* of the activation-deactivation process at the level of insulin sensitive cells.

1. Prager, R., Wallace, P. and Olefsky, J.M. (1986): *J. Clin. Invest.*, 78:472-481.

2. Bergman, R.N., Prager, R., Volund, A., and Olefsky, J.M. (1987). *J. Clin. Invest.*, 79:790-800.

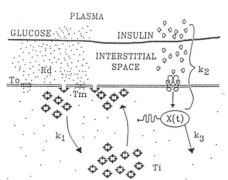

FIG. 1. Model of insulin action. Glucose enters cell in proportion to transporters at membrane. Insulin binds to receptor and increases signal "X(t)". X shuttles transporters to membrane; units return into cell spontaneously. "k" values are kinetic parameters. Parameter k_1 is greater in obese, resulting in less units on membrane at steady-state.

Insulin Action and Diabetes,
edited by H. Joseph Goren et al.
Raven Press, New York © 1988.

ASPECTS OF CLINICAL DISORDERS RELATED TO INSULIN ACTION

Chairman: Dr. D. C. W. Lau

2953, 3330 Hospital Drive. N.W.
Calgary, Alberta
T2N 4N1
The University of Calgary

Intravenous Insulin Self-administration in Diabetic Rats Maintained with Continuous Intravenous or Conventional Subcutaneous Insulin.
E. K. Walls, G. Singer, and T. B. Wishart.

The aim of this study was to determine whether streptozotocin-induced diabetic rats could regulate their own voluntary insulin intake to supplement the different fixed doses of exogenous insulin administered, and whether they could regulate insulin intake when the basal body insulin levels were maintained constant. Rats were trained to receive food pellets and/or insulin by pressing 2 separate levers. In the first series of experiments, voluntary intake of intravenous (iv) insulin was inversely proportional to the fixed subcutaneous (sc) insulin administered daily. Insulin intakes were $0.59+0.09$, $0.48+0.08$, $0.39+0.09$, and $0.23+0.04$ U/day in rats receiving 0, 1, 2, and 4 U Lente insulin sc, respectively. As judged by their food and water intake, and urinary glucose excretion, the insulin self-administering diabetic rats were in better metabolic control than rats receiving only the sc insulin. The second series of studies where diabetic rats were able to self-administer iv insulin in addition to a basal iv infusion showed similar results. The present study suggests that the diabetic rat has the capacity to change its insulin intake appropriately when the basal insulin levels are manipulated.

DISCUSSION

Dr. C. R. Kahn: Could you make a comment how rats did on glucose? Can they sense any reasonable approximation of their glucose and do they attempt to self regulate it?

Dr. E. K. Walls: We actually manipulated carbohydrates and although the rats ate exactly the same amount on each diet the amount of carbohydrates they were given was different.   The amounts of self administered insulin varied according to how much carbohydrates they were given.   Hence the rats were actually responding to the level of glucose induced by dietary carbohydrates.   With a dietary carbohydrate intake of 64% of total energy, the animals were taking about twice as many insulin infusions as they did when the amount of dietary carbohydrate intake was reduced to 33%.

In Vivo and In Vitro Activation of the Rat Muscle Insulin Receptor Kinase.   Effects of Glucocorticoids and Diabetes. N. E. Block and M. G. Buse.   Presented by C. K. Burant

The study was undertaken to examine the molecular mechanisms responsible for the insulin resistance of skeletal muscle in states of hypercortisolemia and insulinopenic diabetes.   Rats were either injected daily with cortisone acetate for 5 days, or given streptozotocin and sacrificed 7 days later.   Insulin receptors were isolated from hindlimb muscle and purified on wheatgerm agglutinin agarose.   Insulin binding to solubilized insulin receptors were studied.   In vitro tyrosine kinase activity was determined by incubating isolated solubilized receptors with poly glu-tyr (4:1) in the absence or presence of increasing insulin concentrations (1-100 nM).   In vivo kinase activity was also assayed. Treatment of rats with glucocorticoids resulted in insulin resistance as evidenced by increased peripheral circulating glucose and insulin levels.   However, glucocorticoids did not alter the insulin binding affinity or number of insulin receptors/cell, or the in vitro and in vivo kinase activation by insulin.   These data suggest that the steroid-induced insulin resistance is likely associated with a post-receptor defect in muscle.   In streptozotocin-induced diabetic rats, insulin receptor binding affinity was unchanged but a 2-fold increase in the receptor number was observed.   Also, the in vivo kinase activation following half-maximal and maximal doses of insulin injection was 40% lower in these animals. Our results are in keeping with the notion that the insulin resistance in diabetes may be explained by impaired activation of the receptor tyrosine kinase.   By examining the insulin stimulated receptor kinase activation in muscle, this model may be applicable to assess insulin resistance in other tissues.

Discussion:

Dr. M. D. Hollenberg: I think it is important to define what you mean by insulin resistance. If it is difficult to dispose of a glucose load the patient is said to be resistent; yet that same patient is very sensitive to insulin in terms of its antilipolytic action.

Dr. C. K. Burant: Clinically insulin resistance is a condition where the insulin level is inappropriately high for any given glucose concentration.

Dr. C. R. Kahn: I think that in certain situations, such as obesity, Type II diabetes, and even steroid treatment in both animals and man, it is pretty clear that there is resistance to insulin action at multiple levels.   In cortisol-treated humans, glucose clamp studies have shown that there is not only a dose response shift to insulin stimulated glucose disposal but also a shift in the dose response to insulin inhibition of glucose output.   Hence insulin resistance occurs at multiple levels. Dr. Zierler in his earlier forearm studies in obese subjects measured multiple responses of insulin, and showed that potassium flux and other things were changed. The only exception is work by Jim Foley in the Pima Indians as they progressively developed Type II diabetes. They actually developed a decreased sensitivity to the insulin effects on glucose transport before they developed resistance to insulin antilipolysis. In other words, resistance to the antilipolytic effect of insulin is absent at a time when there is already some resistance to glucose transport.   That occurs as a phase of the development of the disease and I don't know of any other discordance when one looks at multiple effects.   They really are insulin receptor-mediated effects and not growth-promoting effects or effects mediated by the IGF-I receptor.

Dr. J. Goldman: There is one additional discordance which is truly not an insulin resistent state, and that is the mutant insulin found in a number of families first described by Dr. A. Rubenstein.   These are mutant insulins with decreased biological activity.   The affected subjects usually have hyperinsulinemia and respond normally but they are not insulin resistant.   The hyperinsulinemia is apparently due to the fact that the receptor clearance in the blood is decreased correspondingly.   This is a situation where you could have hyperinsulinemia without insulin resistance and I think it pertains to the comments of Dr. Hollenberg.   If we had a population of molecules of insulin that have decreased biological activity you could conceivably also find hyperinsulinemia without insulin resistance. Maybe we should try to think about alternative ways of finding insulin resistance that in a simple manner could be identified clinically.

Dr. D. A. K. Roncari: I would like to further pursue this discussion on antilipolysis. There is persistence as you know of the antilipolytic effect even in resistance states associated with obesity. Is it because less receptor occupancy is required and then less post binding pathways are required as a consequence? I would like to hear more discussion about this because at the clinical level it is clear that some antilipolysis persists and this may be the reason why ketoacidosis is very rare in diabetes associated with obesity.

Dr. S. W. Cushman: In terms of insulin resistance in general, little attention has been focused on anti-lipolysis and lipid metabolism. I think it is an area in which more attention will need to be paid in the future. I think most people ignore the important relationship between lipid and glucose metabolism that Randall proposed many years ago. There is not yet any evidence to prove that he was wrong. In fact, Gerry Reaven is postulating that a very important mechanism for maintaining hyperglycemia in the diabetic in the basal state is due to an insulin resistance at the level of antilipolysis. A continuous release of fatty acids in the basal state increases substrate availability to the liver and leads to an increase in hepatic glucose production. This will be an area for clarification in the next few years.

Dr. K. Zierler: In the forearm of man if one does insulin response curves, which can't be done as exactly as in vitro, one finds that the responses to insulin with respect to both potassium movement and anti-lipolysis are more sensitive than response to glucose uptake. In other words, you could easily have something that looks like insulin resistance to glucose and still retain the effect of insulin on potassium and on anti-lipolysis. In general, as Dr. Kahn said, when you have obesity and diabetes there is global resistance to insulin.

Effect of Glucose and Insulin on Replication of Cultured Microvascular Endothelial Cells and their Regenerative Response to an Experimental Wound.
D. C. W. Lau, K. L. Wong, and J. M. Forden.

Endothelial injury is a key feature in the early development of diabetic microvascular diseases. Endothelial regeneration which involves cell migration and proliferation may be altered in the diabetic milieu. To evaluate the role of metabolic and hormonal factors in the pathogenesis of diabetic microvascular diseases and retinopathy, we have examined the effects of glucose, insulin, and insulin-like growth factor-I on the growth of rat adipose-tissue-derived (MEC) and bovine retinal microvascular endothelial cells (REC) and their regenerative response to wound injury. An experimental wound was produced by mechanical denudation of a 9-10 mm^2 area of confluent endothelial cells grown on glass coverslips. Cultured rat MEC and bovine REC exposed to high glucose concentrations (12 to 30 mM) both showed significant dose-dependent inhibition in growth as well as their ability to repair wound (p < 0.01 vs control cells grown in 6 mM glucose). High glucose also inhibited retinal pericyte replication in a dose-dependent manner. These observations could not be explained by cell death or extracellular hyperosmolarity since cell viability in all 3 strains was unchanged. Fructose also did not impair wound healing, suggesting that growth inhibition may be mediated through pathways dependent on glucose metabolism, such as the polyol pathway leading to sorbitol production. Insulin (10^{-9} to 10^{-7} M) alone showed a mild inhibition of wound repair whereas in the presence of 18 mM glucose it significantly stimulated the regenerative response, with a maximum effect observed at 10^{-8} M. IGF-I facilitated wound repair at basal and high glucose levels; addition of insulin resulted in a small additional increment in the regenerative response. Our findings in REC were very similar to those observed in MEC, except that the growth rate was slightly slower in REC. The present findings suggest that hyperglycemia may induce endothelial damage and furthermore, retard wound healing. Hyperinsulinemia in the presence of hyperglycemia may accelerate the formation of abnormal new vessels through stimulation of wound repair, which may worsen diabetic microangiopathy and notably, retinopathy. Similarly, IGF-I may also play an important role in the pathogenesis of diabetic vascular diseases.

Discussion:

Dr. C. R. Kahn: Just a quick comment and question. As you know George King at the Joslin Research Laboratories is doing very similar work and has found a very similar effect of glucose on retinal pericytes but not on endothelial cells. The effect on endothelial cells is mimicked by non-metabolizable sugars and appears to be more of an osmotic effect as opposed to a glucose effect whereas in pericytes it requires glucose. I wonder if you compared metabolizable sugars with non-metabolizable sugars to see if these are the same mechanism.

Dr. D. C. W. Lau: Work is currently in progress to address this very important point. The effect of mannitol and other hexoses such as fructose are being examined in detail.

Dr. P. Gorden: If I understand your argument correctly you would say that the major risk, if you were to apply this concept clinically, would be at the time you start intensive insulin therapy whereas when you reach a steady state that risk would be diminished. Is that the implication of your study?

Dr. D. C. W. Lau: What I am advocating is that glycemic control is important in a setting where you have hyperinsulinemia. If we extrapolate from our in vitro data, concomitant hyperglycemia and hyperinsulinemia may aggravate diabetic microvascular complications. In the presence of near normal glycemic control, however, insulin has only a weak mitogenic influence on endothelial cells. The risk for worsening of vascular complications with intensive insulin therapy in the face of euglycemia is low.

Dr. P. Gorden: The question then would really be related to this sort of combined question - should one think about some kind of way to alter intracellular glucose concentrations prior to intense insulin therapy. I don't know that anyone has ever considered that at a time when people are considering intense insulin therapy. Since people are becoming more interested in this form of treatment, I think we have to start thinking about some of the things you are talking about now and ask ourselves questions as to whether there are preparations we need to go through before we institute something like that. Perhaps what Ron Kahn was saying regarding the question of aldose reductase inhibitors or other things prior to the time one would initiate intensive insulin therapy would be something to think about. I wonder if you have thought along those lines and would those be the sort of things you were getting at.

Dr. D. C. W. Lau: That is exactly the point that I am alluding to. It is very important to render poor control to the euglycemic state prior to consideration for intensive insulin therapy. In most situations, as we all know, patients often end up having peripheral hyperinsulinemia, which may indeed aggravate the diabetic vascular complications.

Dr. C. R. Kahn: I would like to comment on the mechanism of hyperglycemic damage. I don't know if you have looked into that, but in these cell cultures the retinal pericytes, again the work of George King, you can show that in a high glucose environment they do accumulate sorbitol and you can block that sorbitol accumulate with aldose reductase inhibitors but that does not reverse the toxic effect of hyperglycemia on cell growth. So that in his hands it is not the mechanism by which hyperglycemia is producing.

Dr. D. C. W. Lau: It has also been shown that hyperglycemia itself can cause DNA damage of endothelial cells. I think that there are a number of possible mechanisms of hyperglycemic damage and what we are proposing here is that hyperinsulinemia coupled with hyperglycemia may accelerate vascular complications. Hence we should be more cautious about intensive insulin therapy in the uncontrolled diabetics.

Insulin Action and Diabetes,
edited by H. Joseph Goren et al.
Raven Press, New York © 1988.

REVIEW OF THE ETIOLOGY OF TYPE I DIABETES
AND OF THE PATHOGENESIS OF ITS COMPLICATIONS

Charles H. Hollenberg M.D.

Banting and Best Diabetes Centre
University of Toronto
3CCRW845, Toronto General Hospital
200 Elizabeth Street
TORONTO, Ontario
Canada   M5G 2C4

Type I diabetes, in which there is an absolute deficiency of insulin, occurs in about 10% of patients with diabetes. Over the last decade enough new information has accumulated about the etiology and outcome of Type I diabetes to allow a general description of the factors which give rise to this particular disease and to some of its complications.

Etiology

Figure 1 is taken from a classic article by George Eisenbarth in The New England Journal of Medicine (3). This figure depicts the current, generally accepted theory as to the etiology of Type I diabetes. There is little doubt but that Type I diabetes develops in individuals who have a genetic predisposition to this disease. Further, it is clear that genetic factors alone are not sufficient to produce diabetes. It is hypothesized that a precipitating event must occur which, in a genetically predisposed individual, incites a variety of immunological responses which, over time, produce a progressive destruction of beta cells, a progressive reduction in insulin release and finally to total absence of endogenous insulin production.

The evidence of genetic predisposition to Type I diabetes is derived from both animal and human data. There are two animal models of Type I diabetes in which the propensity for the development of diabetes is inherited. In the non-obese diabetic mouse the diabetic syndrome is associated with a major histocompatibility gene and, in addition, with at least one other gene outside of the major histocompatiblity complex. In the BB rat the development of diabetes is also genetically linked to a MHC gene and to at least one non-MHC gene. Evidence for genetic susceptibility to Type I diabetes in humans is less direct but nonetheless compelling. Some of these data are summarized in Figure 2. In interpreting the human data it is important to recall that the major histocompatibility genes, located on the short arm of chromosome six, are divided into three classes. Class 1 consists of genes that produce the classical transplant antigens, Class 2 consists of the genes that are responsible for the immune response phenomena, Class 3 are the genes that code for the complement subsets. It is in the group of Class 2 major histocompatibility genes that the link with diabetes has been found. These genes produce antigens that are heterodymeric cell surface glycoproteins. These antigens have a relatively well conserved alpha chain and a variable beta chain. Serological typing of this antigen class has been carried out and a number of antigen sub-sets have been identified. It is the DR sub-sets that are of particular relevance to the etiology of Type I diabetes. Virtually all white patients with Type I diabetes carry the DR3 antigen, the DR4 antigen or both. In heterozygotes who are both DR3 and DR4 positive, the risks are further magnified. In siblings of Type I diabetics who are DR3 or DR4 positive the risk is highest of all. There is also some evidence that in addition to the histocompatibility genes there is at least one other gene locus which is associated with the development of Type I diabetes.

As previously mentioned, Type I diabetes does not develop in all genetically predisposed people. Hence, it is hypothesized that an environmental precipitating event must occur in order for the disease to develop in those who are genetically predisposed. In considering the nature of this precipitating event most attention has been paid to the possibility of viral infection. There is at least one documented case of a Coxsackievirus B_4 being recovered from the pancreas of an individual who died in ketoacidosis soon after the development of Type I diabetes (15). The association of diabetes with congenital rubella has also been recognized for many years. Hence it is possible that, very occasionally, direct virus invasion of the pancreas produces destruction of islet tissue causing Type I diabetes. However if viruses are involved in the development of this disease, it is much more likely that they do so by triggering an autoimmune response which leads to islet cell destruction. There are, of course, many well recognized situations in which infection is followed by auto-immune phenomena. In addition to infection, there may be other environmental factors that incite an autoimmune attack on the pancreas. For example, Dr. Julio Martin has shown that expression of diabetes in the BB rat can be suppressed by removing protein from their diets and feeding them instead an amino acid mixture (4). Whatever the precipitating event, there is now general agreement that in the vast majority of patients with Type I diabetes, the disease occurs as a result of genetic and precipitating factors combining to produce an immune attack on the beta cell.

STAGES IN DEVELOPMENT OF TYPE I DIABETES MELLITUS

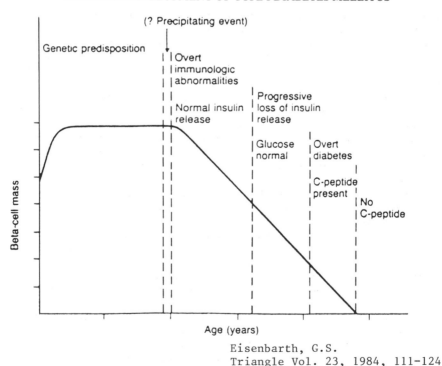

Eisenbarth, G.S.
Triangle Vol. 23, 1984, 111-124

FIG. 1.

ETIOLOGY OF TYPE I DIABETES MELLITUS
HUMAN GENETIC FACTORS

1.	MALE/FEMALE	1.2/1
2.	THYROGASTRIC AUTOANTIBODIES	4 x CONTROL
3.	IDENTICAL TWINS	50% CONCORDANCE
4.	MHC GENES	

ABSOLUTE RISKS

HLA DRx DRx	1 per 5500
DR3 or DR4	1 per 500
DR3 DR3 or DR4 DR4	1 per 125-150
DR3 DR4	1 per 40

PERCENT OF POPULATIONS

DR3 or DR4 or BOTH	CONTROL 40%
	WHITE TYPE 1 95%

5. NON-MHC GENE

FIG. 2.

In considering the role of immunity in the etiology of Type I diabetes, it is useful to turn to the classic article of Gepts in which the pathological anatomy of the pancreas in Type I diabetes is described in great detail (6). While Gepts was not the first to describe luekocytic infiltration of the islets in patients with insulin dependent diabetes, he was the first to indicate the frequency with which this process occurs. Gepts observed this change in 70% of autopsy material from patients with Type I diabetes. Gepts presciently related these histological abnormalities to the possible involvement of an immune process in the development of Type I diabetes. Gepts advanced this hypothesis in 1965, a time when very few individuals were seriously considering the role of autoimmunity in the genesis of diabetes.

Figure 3 sets out some of the data suggesting that autoimmunity is involved in the production of Type I diabetes. In about 70% of patients with recent onset Type I diabetes, antibodies to islet cells can be identified. Indeed, these antibodies are often present many years prior to the overt development of the disease. It is this finding which suggests that the immunological attack on the pancreas proceeds for a long time before beta cell mass is reduced to the point where frank diabetes develops. Amongst non-diabetic individuals islet cell antibodies are found more commonly in those who are first degree relatives of diabetics and who are DR3 or DR4 positive. These data add further evidence of the link between genetic predisposition and autoimmunity in this disorder.

Anti-insulin antibodies can also be detected in high proportion in patients with pre-diabetes and the co-existence of islet cell antibodies and anti-insulin antibodies is a common finding in susceptible individuals. Standardized reagents that will allow anti-islet cell and anti-insulin anti-body reactions to be performed in a reproducible fashion in many laboratories are just becoming available. Obviously, it will be of great interest to use these tests, together with analysis of MHC gene frequency, to identify with some precision population cohorts in whom Type I diabetes is likely to develop.

The final step in the immunological attack upon the beta cell is, of course, the production of activated T cells that invade the beta cells of the pancreas and produce agents, lymphokines, that destroy these cells. The presence of activated T cells has been well documented in diabetic man and diabetic rat and the presence of these cells has been shown to precede the development of the diabetic state. The frequency of activated T cells diminishes after the development of clinical diabetes, presumably because of reduction in the number of functioning islet cells which, in turn, reduces the antigenic stimulus to activated T cell production. There are well documented clinical experiments which indicate that even after a very long period of time, re-exhibition of the beta cell antigen can lead, very quickly, to the reappearance of activated T cells which are beta cell specific. When a pancreatic segmental transplantation was performed, without immunosuppression, from a non-diabetic to a diabetic identical twin, the beta cells of the transplanted pancreas were attacked while the pancreatic segments were not rejected. This led to re-appearance of diabetes in the recipient. This finding indicates that in sensitized individuals the immunological process which produces beta cell destruction and leads to Type I diabetes can be activated very quickly when the appropriate antigenic stimulant is re-applied. These data also suggest that even in pancreatic transplants between identical twins, immunosuppression will be required if beta cells are to survive.

ETIOLOGY OF TYPE I DIABETES MELLITUS PHASE OF ACTIVE IMMUNITY

Anti-islet cell antibodies	— **Positive in 70% of new or pre-diabetics**
	— **Positive in 2% of first degree relatives**
	— **Positive in <0.5% of normal subjects**
	— **High frequency of DR3 or 4**
Anti-insulin antibodies	— **Positive in 30% of pre-diabetics**
	— **Positive in 80% of patients with anti-islet cell antibodies**
Activated T cells	— **precedes diabetes in man & BB rat**

FIG. 3.

Recently studies by Hanahan and his group at Cold Spring Harbour of cell-specific expression of the insulin gene have produced some very interesting data that bear on the etiology of Type I diabetes (8). In these experiments a hybrid gene was produced by annealing the promotor sequence of the insulin gene to another gene whose product could be easily identified. Using microinjection techniques, Hanahan injected this hybrid gene into fertilized mouse embryos at a very early stage of development. The embryos were then placed in the oviducts of pseudopregnant female mice and allowed to develop. A series of transgenic mice were produced which were then mated and a substantial colony of transgenic mice produced. Because the product of the hybrid gene could be readily identified, Hanahan was able to determine with a high degree of precision the cell type in which this hybrid gene was expressed. It was found that the gene product was expressed only in the pancreas and, within that organ, only in the beta cell. Goodman, using similar techniques, has found an identical pattern (12). These studies demonstrate that there exists in the pancreatic beta cell a system which is uniquely capable of turning on, or de-repressing, the insulin gene promotor and, hence, of inducing expression of the gene to which this promotor is fused. Obviously cell specificity with respect to gene expression is controlled through promotor sequences and thus, if gene therapy in Type I diabetes is to work, it will be necessary to fuse the insulin gene with a promotor sequence which can be stimulated in the cell line into which the hybrid gene is injected. Goodman has recently reported some of his early studies in this area (12). Goodman administered cells containing a hybrid gene in which an appropriate promotor sequence was ligated to the insulin gene into immunodeficient diabetic mice. The cells produced insulin in sufficient amounts to lower blood sugar. However, because these cells did not contain the machinery for linking insulin secretion to ambient plasma glucose levels, most of the animals became severely hypoglycemic and died. Hence, while these early experiments in gene therapy of diabetes are of extreme interest, they also highlight the complexity of the problem that confronts the development of appropriate therapy in this area.

To return to the experiments of Hanahan, in following the fate of his transgenic mice, he noted that he could divide these animals into two groups with respect to time of expression of the gene product (1). In one group there was expression of the product of the hybrid gene during embryological or early post-natal life. In this group, presumably because of the induction of immunological tolerance, no autoantibodies to the gene product were produced. In animals in this group, there was no evidence of inflammation in pancreatic islets. However in the second group of transgenic mice, the expression of the gene product was delayed and took place 10 to 12 weeks postpartum. Because of delayed production of the gene product, immunological tolerance could not be induced and autoantibodies were formed to the gene product. Insulitis developed that closely resembled the pattern seen in Type I diabetes. On the basis of these studies, Hanahan hypothesized that a possible cause of autoimmune expression in patients with Type I diabetes is the delayed expression of a gene product. This product could be produced too late in life for the development of immune tolerance and hence the product could incite autoantibody formation and an immunological reaction at the site of production of the protein product. This provocative hypothesis links genetic and autoimmune phenomena in the etiology of Type I diabetes. Obviously its applicability to the human form of insulin dependent diabetes remains to be established.

Immunotherapy of Type I Diabetes

Because of the large body of evidence suggesting that Type I diabetes results from an auto-immune attack on the beta cells of the pancreas, there have been a number of studies both in animals and man of the effects of immunosuppression on the development of Type I diabetes. The data in the animal models are unequivocal. The introduction of immunosuppression at the appropriate time in the biobreeding rat model leads to prevention of the expression of the disease in a high proportion of animals (9). Using the immunosuppressive agent Cyclosporin, a drug which influences T cell function and production, Stiller and his colleagues initiated an open human trial in which Cyclosporin was administered soon after the development of diabetic symptoms in a group of Type I diabetic patients. Stiller found that Cyclosporin administration produced longer and more frequent remissions than would occur otherwise (13). This open trial has now been supplemented by two carefully controlled studies, one in France and a second, a combined study, in Canada and in Europe. The French study has been published (5) and the Canadian/European study has been commented upon at a number of meetings.

In the French study there was randomization of the study group with half being given Cyclosporin, the other half placebo. The entry characteristics of the Cyclosporin and placebo groups were very similar. In this study complete remission was defined as having occurred when, without insulin, the patient achieved a fasting blood sugar of less than 7.8 millimoles per litre, a pc blood sugar of less than 11 millimoles per litre, and a hemoglobin AIC of less than 7.5%. Partial remission was defined as having occurred when a patient achieved these same treatment characteristics with a dose of insulin of .25 units per kilogram per day or less. As shown in Figure 4, administration of Cyclosporin resulted in about one-quarter of the patients remaining in good control without insulin at nine months while less than 10% of the placebo group achieved this result. Cyclosporin treatment also enhanced the frequency of partial remissions. The Canadian study produced very similar results. The Canadian/European study also demonstrated that the response to Cyclosporin was improved if the drug was administered very soon after the appearance of symptoms. In both the French and Canadian studies the major and most worrisome complication of Cyclosporin was elevation of serum creatinine. Fortunately, in both studies, this elevation was mild and was reversed when the Cyclosporin was withdrawn. Other and expected complications included hypertrichosis.

It is important to note that in almost all instances in which Cyclosporin was effective in ameliorating the symptoms and chemical abnormalities of Type I diabetes, withdrawal of Cyclosporin was followed very shortly by recrudescence of diabetic symptoms and hyperglycemia. Hence, to date, there is no evidence that Cyclosporin will permanently turn off the autoimmune attack on the beta cells of the pancreas. The available data all suggest that continuous immunosuppression will be required if the autoimmune process is to be kept in abeyance. This finding is, of course, consonant with the observations related earlier of pancreatic transplants between identical twins.

FRENCH STUDY
INCIDENCE OF REMISSIONS

	CYCLOSPORIN	PLACEBO	p
Complete Remission*			
6 mos.	25% (16 / 63)	19% (11 / 59)	n.s.
9 mos.	24% (13 / 54)	6% (3 / 52)	<0.01
Complete & Partial Remission			
6 mos.	46% (29 / 63)	29% (17 / 59)	0.05
9 mos.	37% (20 / 54)	16% (7 / 52)	<0.01

* Blood Glucose <7.8 mM / L

FIG. 4. (5)

In addition to immunosuppression, there is another form of experimental therapy in Type I diabetes which is currently being explored. This therapy involves segmental pancreatic transplantation, almost always done at the time of renal transplantation in patients with diabetic renal disease. Figure 5 sets out a historical view of the success of pancreatic transplantation in patients with Type I diabetes. Obviously, with time, not only have the number of pancreatic transplants increased but the instances of graft survival have also increased. However, at the present time, despite these advances, when pancreatic transplantation and renal transplantation are done together, the mortality rate associated with renal transplantation alone is doubled. Hence there continues to be a very substantial mortality associated with pancreatic transplantation. Nonetheless there are several surgical centers that are pursuing this particular mode of treatment vigorously and with every expectation of significant improvement in both graft survival and in mortality.

Other approaches to treatment of Type I diabetes have involved transplantation of pancreatic islets rather than of whole pancreatic segments. Dr. Tony Sun at Connaught Laboratories has pioneered in an attempt to achieve successful transplantation of islets by encapsulating the islets in alginate-polylysine membranes. Dr. Sun has achieved some success with this particular approach although it appears that the microcapsules do not prevent the development of an immune response.

PANCREAS TRANSPLANTATION

ERA	NO. OF TRANSPLANTS	ONE YEAR PATIENT SURVIVAL	ONE YEAR GRAFT SURVIVAL
1966-77	64	40%	3%
1978-82	201	72%	20%
1983-86	565	78%	41%

FIG. 5.

Pathogenesis of Complications of Type I Diabetes

Recent expansion of knowledge in the etiology and treatment of Type I diabetes has been accompanied by a considerable growth in our understanding of the mechanisms by which some of the long term complications of the disease are produced. In this area there are three developments of particular interest. The first has been the demonstration that the non-enzymatic glycosylation of proteins which occurs in an accelerated fashion in diabetes is associated with the microvascular complications of the disease. The second has been the demonstration that Type I diabetes is associated with an alteration in microvascular hemodynamics within the kidney and that repair of this abnormality can prevent some of the renal abnormalities associated with diabetes. Thirdly, it has been demonstrated that Type I diabetes is associated with abnormalities of polyinositol metabolism in peripheral nerve and that these abnormalities can be associated with some of the neuropathic changes seen in diabetes.

Several years ago Monnier demonstrated that collagen solubilized from skin biopsies of normal and diabetic subjects would fluoresce when excited (10, 11). This fluorescence is caused by cross-linking of collagen fibrils which results from the non-enzymatic glycosylation of the collagen fibril. The cross-linking is due to linkages between the carbohydrate residues. The data in Figure 6 taken from Monnier indicates that this fluorescence is progressive with age and proceeds more rapidly in diabetic subjects than in non-diabetic controls. Extrapolation of the two lines in the figure show that they intersect at 11 years of age, the average time of onset of diabetes in the diabetic subjects. These data suggest that glycosylation of collagen occurs at a constant rate in both the diabetic and non-diabetic subjects but more rapidly in the former. Figure 7 analyzes the data with respect to the presence or absence of retinopathy and according to the degree of severity of retinopathy. In patients without retinopathy the rate of progress of glycosylation and cross-linking is no different than in the control population. However, in patients with either Grade 1 or Grade 2 retinopathy the rate of development of collagen cross-linking is two to three times more rapid than in the control group. These data indicate a relationship between cross-linking of collagen fibrils and the development of a significant complication of diabetes. Those patients in whom the rate of cross-linking was not different from control did not develop this particular diabetic complication. Experimentally, cross-linking of collagen fibrils can be prevented by administration of amino-guanidine. Aminoguanidine links to the reactive carbonyl on the carbohydrate residue which is responsible for cross-linkage phenomenon. Administration of aminoguanidine to diabetic rats has been shown to prevent diabetes-induced formation of fluorescence, in this instance in arterial wall connective tissue protein (2). Demonstration that this compound can prevent the cross-linking of collagen associated with non-enzymatic glycosylation opens an interesting avenue of study as to the significance of protein glycosylation in the production of diabetic complications.

EFFECT OF AGE ON COLLAGEN FLUORESCENCE

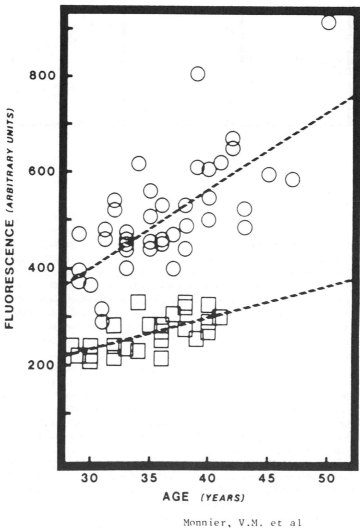

Monnier, V.M. et al
JClinInvest. Vol.78 1986,832

FIG. 6. OPEN CIRCLES - DIABETICS, SQUARES - CONTROLS

COLLAGEN FLUORESCENCE AND RETINOPATHY

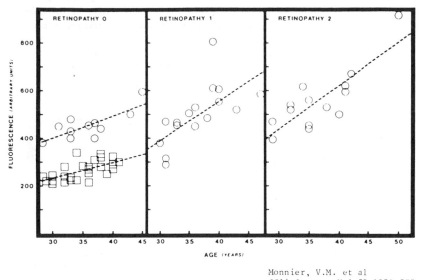

Monnier, V.M. et al
JClinInvest. Vol.78,1986,832

FIG. 7. OPEN CIRCLES - DIABETICS, SQUARES - CONTROLS

In addition to diabetic retinopathy, diabetic glomerulosclerosis is another microvascular complication of diabetes. In a series of elegant studies from Brenner's laboratory (16) it was shown that experimental diabetes in rats produces glomerular hyperfiltration which is due to an increase in gradient and pressure across the glomerular membrane. The increase in gradient in diabetes results from changes in resistance in the efferent relative to the afferent arteriole. Glomerular hypertension produces glomerulosclerosis which can be graded pathologically. When an angiotensin 1 converting enzyme inhibitor is administered to diabetic rats, the enzyme inhibitor has no effect on metabolic control but lowers systemic blood pressure, improves microvascular hemodynamics, and prevents pathological renal change. The enzyme inhibitor reduces transglomerular hydraulic pressure by altering arteriolar resistance within the kidney. Since the enzyme inhibitor has no effect on metabolic control, the effect of the enzyme inhibitor on this particular complication of diabetes results entirely from hemodynamic alterations. In a related study Brenner and his collaborators found that the converting enzyme inhibitor also lessens another manifestation of diabetic renal injury, microalbuminuria. These studies offer compelling evidence that manipulation of factors that control glomerular hypertension might be very important in determining the pace of development of diabetic glomerulosclerosis.

The third area of research which has led to new concepts in the etiology of diabetic complications relates to the role of derangements in phosphoinositol metabolism in the development of diabetic neuropathy. A number of years ago Winegrad and his collaborators proposed that hyperglycemia produces accumulation of sorbitol in tissues which in turn reduces the tissue level of myo-inositol leading to an impairment of nerve conduction (14). More recent studies have provided a more complete picture of the link between hyperglycemia and abnormal nerve conduction. Figure 8, taken from a recent article by Green and his collaborators (7), summarizes recent concepts in this area.

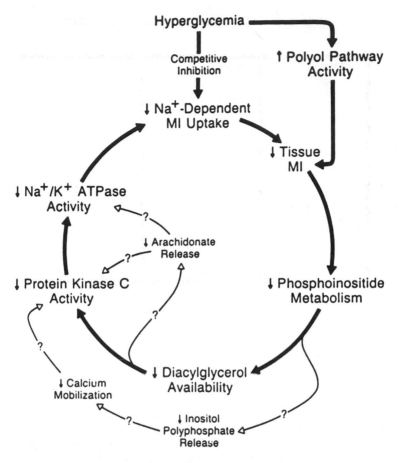

FIG. 8. SORBITOL PATHWAY & PHOSPHOINOSITIDE METABOLISM   (7).
Reprinted by permission of *The New England Journal of Medicine* (316:599–606, 1987).

Hyperglycemia induces activation of the polyol pathway because of conversion of intracellular glucose to sorbitol by the enzyme aldose reductase. The activation of the polyol pathway produces a reduction in tissue myo-inositol. Reduced tissue levels of myo-inositol reduce the turnover of phosphoinositol which in turn results in a decreased intracellular availability of diacyl glycerol. Since diacyl glycerol activates protein kinase C, reduced availability of diacyl glycerol limits protein kinase C activation. This, in turn, reduces the activity of sodium-potassium-ATPase. Reduced sodium-potassium-ATPase activity leads to an increase in sodium content in nerve, particularly around the nodes of Ranvier leading to nerve swelling and decreased nerve conduction. It is also likely that decreased sodium-potassium-ATPase activity interferes with sodium dependent uptake of myo-inositol leading to further depletion of tissue myo-inositol levels and reinforcement of the metabolic defect. Experimentally, the administration of aldose reductase inhibitors or administration of myo-inositol can elevate diacyl glycerol levels and hence increase protein kinase C activity leading to a restoration of nerve conduction. Clinical trials of aldose reductase inhibitors are underway but the results to date have been equivocal.

Despite these very significant advances in our understanding of the pathogenesis of diabetic complications, there still remains the very significant question as to whether control of diabetic hyperglycemia can lead to a reduction in diabetic complications. In order to answer this question once and for all, a multi-centre diabetes control and complications trial has been initiated by the National Institutes of Health. This trial involves approximately 1400 people with Type I diabetes, half in a standard treatment group and half in an experimental group. The standard treatment group is given insulin twice daily while the experimental group is treated either by continuous infusion of insulin or by three or more injections of insulin per day. It is already clear that these two treatment regimes produce very different degrees of glycemic control. The end point of the study is the development or worsening of diabetic retinopathy. The trial is now several years old and it is planned that it will continue for another six to seven years. This trial should provide definitive data as to whether rigourous diabetic control can affect the development of the microvascular complications of diabetes.

Summary

It is now considered likely that Type I diabetes is an autoimmune disease which occurs in genetically predisposed individuals. Hypothetical environmental triggering factors set off the autoimmune response which, over time, results in destruction of islet cells. Administration of immunosuppressive agents soon after the onset of diabetic symptoms can result, in some, in a suppression of the immune attack on islet cells but this attack resumes when the immunosuppressive agents are removed. Recent studies on the pathogenesis and complications of diabetes suggests that it is likely that hyperglycemia has a direct influence on the development of both the retinal and neurological complications of this disease. A long term, large scale human study of the effectiveness of close diabetic control on diabetic complications is underway.

References

1. Adams, T.E., Alpert, S. and Hanahan, D. (1987): Nature, 325:223-228
2. Brownlee, M., Vlassara, H., Kooney, A., Ulrich, P. and Cerami, A. (1986): Science, 232:1629-1632
3. Eisenbarth, G.S. (1986): N.Engl.J.Med., 314:1360-1368
4. Elliott, R.B. and Martin, J.M. (1984): Diabetologia, 26:297-299
5. Feutren, G., Papoz, L., Assan, R., Vialettes, B., Karsenty, G., Vexiau, P., DuRostu, H., Rodier, M., Sirmai, J., Lallemand, A. and Bach, J.-F. (1986): Lancet 2:119-124
6. Gepts, W. (1965): Diabetes, 14:619-633
7. Greene, D.A., Lattimer, S.A. and Sima, A.A.F. (1987): N.Engl.J.Med., 316:599-606
8. Hanahan, D. (1985): Nature, 315:115-122
9. Laupacis, A., Stiller, C.R., Gardell, C., Keown, P., Dupre, J., Wallace, A.C. and Thibert, P. (1983): Lancet, 1:10-15
10. Monnier, V.M., Elmets, C.A., Frank, K.E., Vishwanath, V. and Yamashita, T. (1986): J.Clin. Invest., 78:832-835
11. Monnier, V.M., Vishwanath, V., Frank, K.E., Elmets, C.A., Dauchot, P. and Kohn, R.R. (1986): N.Engl.J.Med., 314:403-408
12. Selden, R.F., Skoskiewicz, M.J., Russell, P.S. and Goodman, H.M. (1987): N.Engl.J.Med., 317:1067-1076
13. Stiller, C.R., Dupre, J., Gent, M., Jenner, M.R., Keown, P.A., Laupacis, A., Martell, R., Rodger, N.W., Graffenried, B.v. and Wolfe, B.M.J. (1984): Science, 223:1362-1367
14. Winegrad, A.I., Greene, D.A. (1976): N.Engl.J.Med., 295:1416-1421
15. Yoon, J.W., Austin, M., Onodera, T. and Notkins, A.L. (1979): N.Engl. J. Med., 300:1173-1179
16. Zatz, R., Rentz Dunn, B., Meyer, T.W., Anderson, S., Rennke, H.G. and Brenner, B.M. (1986): J.Clin.Invest., 77:1925-1930

Insulin Action and Diabetes,
edited by H. Joseph Goren et al.
Raven Press, New York © 1988.

INSULIN ACTION AND DIABETES: EPILOGUE AND PROLOGUE

Morley D. Hollenberg

Endocrine Research Group, Dept. of Pharmacology & Therapeutics
University of Calgary, Faculty of Medicine
Calgary, Alberta, T2N 4N1

It may be difficult, if not impossible, in the area of
diabetes-related research, to recreate the kind of excitement
engendered by the dramatic therapeutic effects of insulin, when
first used in the early 1920's for patients like Leonard
Thompson. Understandably, at that time many must have thought
that the cure for diabetes was well in hand. Yet, at this
conference, held more than 60 years after the discovery of
insulin, we must admit that we really don't know exactly how
insulin works; and we aren't even sure about the best way to
use insulin in diabetics of either the Type I or Type II
classification. This situation of relative ignorance is both
challenging and sobering for us all. Yet, the kind of information that has been shared at this conference on Insulin Action
and Diabetes, and that has been summarized in this volume,
represents a new wave of excitement that bears not only on the
pathophysiology of diabetes itself, but also on other disorders,
such as cancer, which may involve functional derangements of
receptors, like the one for insulin, that exhibit tyrosine
kinase activity. In many ways, the topics presented here are
representative of a new research threshold. By way of an
epilogue for the conference, one can point with great enthusi-
asm to some of the first public discussions about the intimate
anatomic details of the insulin receptor per se: about the
precise receptor amino acid sequence; about the necessity of
its intrinsic tyrosine kinase activity for generating a biological response; about the variety of sites of phosphorylation
that are triggered when insulin binds; and about the complex
receptor dynamics, both at the cell surface and upon internalization, that ensue when insulin binds to the receptor. Thus,
some of the initial molecular events related to insulin action
are in the process of being documented.

But, after insulin binds and activates the receptor, what
happens next? As summarized in this volume, insulin causes a
myriad of cellular effects; and the time course of 'what
happens next' ranges from milliseconds (changes in membrane

243

potential), to minutes (regulation of glucose transport) to hours or tens of hours (regulation of gene expression). Thus, it may come as no surprise that the search for mediators of insulin action is focussing on a variety of potential candidates ranging from a number of intriguing phosphoproteins, thought to be targets for the receptor kinase, to several complex membrane-derived glycophospholipids. The mechanisms whereby these multiple putative mediators of insulin action modulate cell function remain a subject of intense enquiry; and the growing understanding of transmembrane signalling mechanisms, discussed informally during the conference, provides just cause to be optimistic that the precise biochemical links between receptor occupation and cell activation by insulin will be forged in the very near future.

Nonetheless, despite the narrowing of the gap in knowledge between the events of receptor occupation and cell activation, a wide gap still remains between this newly-found knowledge and its practical application for the treatment of diabetic patients. However, in this area as well, as indicated by several presentations at this conference, there is cause for modest optimism. For instance, the recently acquired information about the structure and tyrosine kinase activity of the receptor has generated new perspectives for understanding and diagnosing insulin resistance at the level of the receptor; and the new understanding of receptor dynamics and insulin-triggered receptor regulation has had a direct practical impact upon insulin dosing regimens used in a variety of clinical settings. Interestingly, developments in understanding membrane receptor function and receptor-triggered transmembrane signalling reactions are providing new insights for the understanding of the possible consequences to membrane function of hyperglycemia per se, and for the understanding of the precise mechanisms whereby autoimmune processes lead to pancreatic beta cell destruction. These new insights, and the prospective clinical trials that these new insights have generated will have a direct impact on the care and treatment of diabetic patients in the future.

Thus, this epilogue for what has been a most exciting conference on Insulin Action and Diabetes is also a Prologue for what is to come. The signposts of what is to come have been solidly planted; and there is an ever-growing conviction that we are on the right track to understanding diabetic pathophysiology. It is with great anticipation that we all look forward to new developments in this highly rewarding area of biomedical research; and it will be with considerable interest and amusement that we will all look back at the proceedings of this conference to determine if the discoveries made during this time period really do represent the same kind of watershed for diabetes-related research typified by the discovery of insulin.

Subject Index

A

Acetyl-CoA carboxylase regulation, 173–184
Acidification, 142
Activation model, 148
Adenosine triphosphate (ATP)
  binding of
    autophosphorylation, 44
    mutagenesis, 52
    human insulin receptor, 1
    insulin receptor autophosphorylation sites, 54–55
    insulin receptor kinase and, 43,44
    tyrosine kinases and, 3
Adipocyte(s)
  cellular target site, 117–128
  insulin action, 92–102
  insulin-, isoproterenol-, and phorbol ester-treated, 157–162
  mediator substances, 107,109
  phospholipase C activation by insulin in, 113–115
  subcellular distribution of insulin receptor tyrosine kinase activity in, 151–156
Adipose tissue, acetyl-CoA carboxylase activity and, 173–174,177–182
Alanine, endosomal kinase activity, 143
Alpha–beta heterodimers. *See* Functional alpha–beta heterodimers
Alpha subunit (insulin receptor); *see also* Beta subunit; Insulin receptor
  composition of, 43
  endosomal kinase activity, 148
  linkage of, 73
Amino acid(s); *see also* Peptides
  beta subunit, 44
  human insulin receptor, 1,2
  identification of Tyr(P) in sequence analysis of, 67–71
  insulin receptor autophosphorylation sites, 56–57,60
Aminoguanidine, 238
AMP concentrations, 174
Antigens. *See* Class I transplantation antigens

Antiphosphotyrosine immunoaffinity chromatography, 56,60
Antiphosphotyrosine monoclonal antibodies, 62–63
Anti-receptor antibody, 35,36
ASD-insulin, 30–31
ATP. *See* Adenosine triphosphate
ATZ-Tyr(P), 67–71
Autophosphorylation; *see also* Phosphorylation
  activation of, 119
  adipocytes, 152–156
  beta subunit, 53–54,185–187
  cell surface insulin receptor, 38–40
  cellular target and, 117
  endosomal kinase activity, 142–143, 145,149
  insulin-dependent beta subunit, 84–85
  insulin effect, 78
  insulin receptor tyrosine residues identification *in vitro* and *in vivo*, 53–66
  monoclonal antibodies, 53–54
  monomers, 79–80
  protein, 129
  receptor tyrosine kinase activation, 61–64
  site location, 43–52
  tyrosine kinase, 43
Avidin, 23

B

Beta cell(s), 235
Beta subunit; *see also* Alpha subunit; Insulin receptor
  autophosphorylation site, 43–52,84–85,185–187
  composition of, 43
  endosomal kinase activity, 142,143
  identification of [32P]Tyr(P) on multiple phosphorylated peptides from, 67–72
  insulin receptor autophosphorylation sites, 54,57,59,60
  linkage of, 73